# COVENTRY LIBRARIES

Please return this book on or before
the last date stamped below.

D1348155

To renew this book take it to any of
the City Libraries before
the date due for return

# What can i do to Help?

**75 PRACTICAL IDEAS FOR FAMILY AND FRIENDS FROM CANCER'S FRONTLINE**

## Deborah Hutton

First published in 2005 by
Short Books
3A Exmouth House
Pine Street
London EC1R 0JH

This paperback edition published in 2010
10 9 8 7 6 5 4 3 2

A CIP catalogue record for this book
is available from the British Library.

978-1-906021-56-6
Printed and bound by
CPI Group (UK) Ltd, Croydon, CR0 4YY
Jacket design: Emily Fox

## Acknowledgements

Books like this are never the work of just one person. First and foremost, thanks to those, known and not so well known, who generously contributed their insights and experiences. Big thanks too to Clare Alexander, Paris Back, Maggie Bisset, Sarah Caplin, P and Martin Fiennes, Gill Haines, Marianna Falconer, Rebecca Nicolson at Short Books, who ran with the idea from its inception, Demelza Short and the 18 Highbury 'Colander Girls', Helen Simpson, Jennifer Thompson and, last but not least, my fabulous family – Charlie, already known throughout north London as the sainted one, and my four children who, showing a maturity beyond their years, put their own needs aside at the toughest of times and allowed this project to take precedence.

When we first had the idea of approaching high-profile names and asking them to contribute examples for the book, it was not without reservations. My experience as a journalist had taught me that approaching such people is generally a heart-sinking round of put-offs, prevarications and flat refusals. Not so in this case. In 2005, cancer may still be the disease that cannot speak its name, but it is also the great leveller – cutting across divisions of class, income, status and success – and, sadly, so ubiquitous that few people's lives are untouched by it. Almost without exception, those we approached gave their time and reminiscences not only with great open-heartedness but with touching concern for my own welfare. They were…

Clive Anderson, Tony Benn, Cherie Blair, Alastair Campbell, Richard Chartres (the Bishop of London), Sir Colin Davis, Monty Don, Lord Falconer (the Lord Chancellor), Dawn French, Duncan Goodhew, Jade Goody, Hugh Grant, Loyd Grossman, Patricia Hodge, Nicola and Alice Horlick, Gloria Hunniford, Sir Elton John, Felicity Kendal, Tessa Jowell, Maureen Lipman, Joanna Lumley, Miriam Margolyes, Mo Mowlam, Rabbi Julia Neuberger, Esther Rantzen, Corin Redgrave, Anne Robinson, Gaby Roslin, Nick Ross, Nigel Slater, Jon Snow, Ruby Wax, Bob Wilson and Sam Taylor-Wood.

# Contents

Introduction 9

Immediately after the diagnosis 21

What should I say? 69

During treatment 97

Practicalities 122

Searching… 151

When the going gets tough 173

Survivorship 214

About Macmillan 238

Information 244

Bibliography 253

# Introduction

I count myself the luckiest and unluckiest woman in London. The luckiest because I have a great husband, a fabulous family with kids on track and growing up, a beautiful house, more friends than I deserve and as much interesting work as I want. This time a year ago, I'd put the dog on the lead and walk over to the local shops in the sunshine marvelling at my own good fortune, thinking I wouldn't swap places with anyone in the world.

Then, at a stroke, this lovely run of luck ran out. On 26 November 2004, at the age of 'just' 49 and a half, which my kids think is ancient but seems pretty young to me, I discovered that the irritating, niggly cough I had had for the past two months was no trivial chest infection but an aggressive adenocarcinoma that had already spread well beyond the organ of origin – my lungs – to my bones, lymph nodes and possibly my liver as well.

The irony of my situation was apparent to everyone who knew me. I was the healthiest woman on the block: never ill, never down, a runner of half-marathons, and a yoga freak and nutrition nut to boot. I knew how to look after myself big time. After all, it was my job. I had been writing about women's health for more than a quarter of a century, first as health editor of *Vogue* and then for a range of glossy magazines and newspapers. I was the published author of not one but four books about preventive health. Since giving up smoking 23 years ago, I had joined the ranks of those fanatically intolerant anti-smoking ex-smokers. And yet here I now was struck down by lung cancer, with its serves-you-right stigma.

Faced with the facts of my unenviable situation, it was hard not to feel incredulous. I looked like a well woman – and with the exception of the cough, and the recurrent one-sided headaches, and the pain in my left hip, and the three-quarters of a stone that had unaccountably tumbled off since September, I felt a well woman. How could I have a stage IV cancer that, even now, was racing round my body, invading my vital organs, threatening to kill me? And quite soon by all accounts. 'Don't look up your cancer on the internet,' my consultant warned me just before backing out of my side-room at University College Hospital. 'You'll only terrify yourself.' I didn't, but even so it didn't take long to find out that in the distinctly unwonderful world of advanced cancer, stage IV is as bad as it gets. There is no stage V.

It was the worst of all news – 'as bad as it can get,' confirmed the nurse at the Middlesex Hospital who rang to inform me that the CT scan had revealed mets (= metastases = spread) in my liver. Was there anywhere that this cancer wasn't? And yet, though I was reeling from the discovery that few of my vital organs seemed to be free of this thing, I didn't feel my luck had entirely run out. Even then, I continued to count myself fortunate. How so?

Well, I had the highest level of support imaginable. I would look at my companions in the Middlesex chemo suite, alone and unsupported, undergoing their notoriously tough treatments and then having to find their own way home at the end of them, and I felt extraordinarily blessed. I happen to be married to one of the most remarkable men on the planet – the kindest, funniest, most generous, emotionally intelligent human being in existence, who seems to have been assembled (correctly!) from a *New Man* catalogue and who makes me laugh more than anyone else I know. We have four gorgeous and exceptionally warm-hearted children, aged eight, 11, 14 and 17 on the day of diagnosis. Fanning out from there, in both directions, we are lucky enough to have large close-knit families, including in my case a twin sister, non-identical, who dropped everything immediately and raced up to be with me.

Add a world-class network of friends and neighbours, who were determined from the outset to save me so much as a second of unnecessary stress or strain, and Marvellous Maggie, the palliative care nurse who was allocated to me following my very first clinic appointment. From the outset, she has taken my welfare, physical and emotional, to heart, regularly ringing me, always prefacing her call with 'Is this a good time?', organising my pain relief, coming to see me and, in her calm, reassuring tones, answering all my questions as well as those of my children, whom she has also taken under her wing. Factor in all of this, and you will see that I was actually in the world's best possible position to receive the world's worst possible news.

Before the week was out, for example, a supper rota had been set up by one mover and shaker in our north London street, sparing me the hassle of thinking or planning or shopping or cooking for my family. Knowing how quickly the best intentions can dissolve in the face of the demands of a busy life – all these women, whom I have taken to calling the 'Colander Girls', have families to raise, and most have jobs to juggle, too – it amazes me that, six months on, they are still dishing up their delicacies and that more are requesting to join the rota every month. At the time of writing, they now number 18.

Back then, the idea was inspired. If I was in shock, and quite unable to know what to do or where to turn, my friends and family were too. 'Shocked', 'devastated', 'numb', 'disbelieving' – these were the adjectives that came up again and again in the avalanche of letters and cards arriving by every post, the flowers and gifts and phone calls we received at all hours of the day, every day. While this outpouring of love and concern was wonderfully uplifting, it was also bone-crushingly wearying. In fact, it soon became clear that if the cancer didn't finish me off sharpish, the telephone most certainly would. It rang and rang until we almost started hearing it in our sleep.

At the same time, I recognised that calls had to be taken and visits received. Friends and family needed the reassurance of seeing me and/or hearing my voice, still clear and strong, and to realise that, even though I was now under a sudden and most unexpected sentence of death, I was still very much with them. Most of all, they yearned to do something, anything, to help, to feel useful not useless, to support us in whatever way they could. 'It is not easy to work out how we who know you and love you, and who luckily do not have cancer as far as we know, can help,' wrote one close friend, soon after the diagnosis. 'We know sometimes what to do. We know sometimes what not to do. Mostly we stumble around in the dark and try, crossing our fingers that whatever it is will prove right and not horribly wrong for you.'

Even though I recognised from the outset that I was amazingly privileged, it took a while to accept the help in the spirit it was offered. I have always been the one who prefers to be 'in credit' – whether by doing an extra school run or cooking the supper. A super-energetic – some have called me manic – organising type, it's always been second nature to me to say, 'No, I'll do it' or 'Come to us' or 'This one's on me'. Suddenly, the tables were turned, and I was overwhelmed by the number of people now queuing up to do something for me. As the initial panicky sense of having the carpet rudely whipped from under my feet subsided and we adapted to this very unwelcome visitor in our midst, I found myself at the beginning of a brand-new learning curve. I had to let go of years of pride in being so capable and tough and self-reliant, to accept how wonderful it might be to shed some of my responsibilities and let others take them on, and to begin to learn about life on the receiving end.

It wasn't easy. After 30 years of independence, I found I had a nameless dread of what might happen if I was not there holding it all together. I had such an iron grip on all the minutiae of family life, I was terrified that if I let go for so much as a single second, the whole thing would implode. If I accepted the help on offer, would I ever recover my coping skills? Would I ever be able to put supper on the table or drive the children anywhere again? After just four days in hospital, I had already begun to feel institutionalised. This was in itself scary. Like so many women, I suspect, I felt like I was a vessel containing all the emotional and practical needs of everyone in the family, right down to the dog and cats and even the goldfish. If I foundered on the rocks and went down, then they would, too.

In the event, I discovered it was a tremendous relief to be able to let go, to allow my friends to take the strain, whether it was doing some of the Christmas shopping and present-wrapping, or taking on phone calls and ballet runs. It taught me that life would and could go on, if a bit bumpily, without my overseeing presence; a good rehearsal, you might say, for my ultimate departure. It also taught me that it can be extraordinarily good for the other members of a family – particularly one with such a managerial mother – to develop their own areas of competence and to feel that they themselves can contribute something of real value in a crisis.

Allowing myself to be supported in many of the myriad ways outlined in this book also helped those friends and extended family members who were standing on the sidelines, wringing their hands and wondering what they could do. To begin with, my impulse was to say, 'No, no I'm fine. We're managing. Don't worry.' But then I realised that this was helping no one – not me, still in shock, nor those around me who were feeling just as devastated and helpless. They were quite desperate to help, to do something, anything, to relieve their sense of powerlessness.

By putting that super-competent, I-can-handle-it-myself-thank-you-very-much persona aside and learning to say, 'Yes,

I'd like that, thank you' or 'You know you said absolutely anything – well, do you think you could possibly…?', I began to understand that I was actually helping them. I learned to accept their offers gratefully and graciously – whether it was scooping up the children, or cooking Wednesday night's supper, or driving me to one of the endless hospital appointments and sitting alongside me in the grim clinics while we waited to see yet another registrar or consultant to bash us with yet another bout of bad news, or snuggling up under the duvet and companionably watching a DVD on a weekday afternoon.

'How many of us, how often, have come out with the banal "Do just let me know if there's anything I can do" or "If only there was something I could do",' asked Sooze, an old friend of mine, on my blog, the interactive internet diary that I set up a fortnight after my diagnosis. 'And how many of us have ever had instant take-up with "Yes" followed by a litany of tasks?

'No, far more likely that we'll spend a while in the card shop, ring up the florist to despatch the token plant, and ask others from time to time how you are getting on. Abdication big time. Giving me something I could actually do for you that was easily accomplished and gave pleasure and cost nothing [in her case cheering me up by contributing frequent, funny and irreverent comments to the blog] helped me every bit as much as you – even more so, perhaps.'

Over a quarter of a million people are diagnosed with cancer every year in the UK. The statisticians at Macmillan

Cancer Relief have worked out that this means 739 people receive the worst piece of news imaginable every day, unexpectedly finding themselves members of the last club in the world they would ever choose to join. The Cancer Club. The only club I can think of that is both rigorously exclusive and has no waiting list. Ever. At the beginning, I shrank from identification with its sad membership: the embattled, the brave and the bald. But actually I found amazing solace and shining acts of generosity there.

Women who were friends of friends, or even friends of friends of friends, helpfully passed on their tips, told me what had sustained them in the dark days after the diagnosis; what had helped and what had hindered. One woman, also diagnosed with cancer in her lungs and bones, but 18 months previously, rejigged her social arrangements at the last minute to come and pick our shell-shocked family off the floor the evening after we had broken the news to them. For them to see a living, breathing, *well* person coming through the door, looking fabulous, and chatting and answering their questions before nipping off to a dinner party elsewhere, did more to lift their spirits than any amount of reassurance we could have provided.

While this was well timed and fantastically supportive, the truth is that some forms of 'help', however well intentioned, can be more debilitating than the after-effects of chemotherapy. Like what? 'Like the constant phone calls asking

17

how you are, which means continually updating everyone on how you're feeling and how the treatment's going, until you could weep from weariness,' said one woman. (A problem I got round by setting up the blog and posting regular reports. Directing well-wishers to an internet address saved hours of repetitious conversations for which I simply didn't have the energy or inclination.)

'Like people I didn't know very well ringing and bursting into tears down the phone – I could have really done without that,' said another friend who, like so many people newly diagnosed with cancer, found herself having to deal with other people's fear and shock and grief when she herself was wrestling with the same emotions tenfold. Even the best-intentioned advice can impose additional burdens. 'Those endless people telling you that you absolutely MUST see this marvellous herbalist/acupuncturist/healer in Southend or Mexico or Timbuktu.'

My hope is that this book will help you, and new members of the Cancer Club, to identify the need and to ask for/provide it. Despite sharing the 'same' disease (in fact, there are more than 200 different types of malignancy, which geneticists are now saying may subdivide into as many as 2,000), we are all different – both in how we react and in what we require. Nevertheless, there are some common threads that will help you to be on the side of the angels and to avoid some of the pitfalls that await the unwary (into which I, in my previously healthy incarnation, now realise I fell many times).

As a person living with cancer, I would never presume to know what anyone else needs. I am just passing on aspects of my experience and that of the hundreds of others I have spoken to in the course of my research for this book. The key, I quickly found, is to zero in on everyone's strengths and to build on them: ask the car drivers to take you places, the conscientious mothers to scoop up your children, the cordon bleu cooks to provide an evening meal, the good Christians (or Jews or Muslims or Buddhists) to pray for your healing and recovery. Ask friends whose intellect and judgement you respect to comb the internet for information on everything from cutting-edge new clinical trials to wacky-sounding alternative remedies, while screening out the unpalatable facts such as survival and/or treatment rates if they present more reality than you feel you can take. Allow your good friends to act as gatekeepers of your diary, to keep visits at a manageable level, to field phone calls and to work out a rota of who will accompany you to hospital appointments, chemo or radiotherapy sessions, kidney or bone scans.

Flowers and plants, lovely and cheering as they are, soon fade and die, and visits can be wearying, but help with the practicalities is an ongoing joy. The grim reality of cancer, and any other serious illness, is that life, with all its demands, continues: the children still need transporting to and from school, the dog needs walking, the laundry needs ironing and the daily meals need planning, preparing and dishing up. These every-day tasks can feel overwhelmingly burdensome when you are feeling shell-shocked and are trying to fit them around the myriad visits to clinics and specialists that follow in the wake of every cancer diagnosis.

'What can I do to help?' you ask. Well, stand by, because the answer is: plenty.

# Immediately after the diagnosis

A diagnosis of cancer changes everything: how we feel about ourselves, our health, our relationships, our livelihood and means of supporting our families, our future. In this new and unfamiliar landscape, we are suddenly no longer the fit, capable people we may have thought we were – but sick, weakened, frail mortals under siege from a disease whose very name still conjures an unholy terror among many of the people about us and from thoughts of frightening future possibilities.

*It felt like the universe turned into a thin paper tissue, and then someone simply tore the tissue in half right in front of my eyes.* Treya Killam Wilber, *Grace and Grit*

*I thought, cancer doesn't happen to me. It's not in my family. I've always looked after myself. It can't happen to me.* Nazira Visram

*The doctor went on talking, but once he'd said the word 'cancer' I was in such shock I couldn't hear the words coming out of his mouth.* Dee Dee Hope

*It felt like my life had changed in a minute for ever. I felt devastated for a long, long time.* Anna Blackman

Even if we are one of the lucky unlucky ones and ours is a stage I cancer, with every hope of a complete cure, the news still comes like a thump in the solar plexus, especially if the diagnosis is unexpected. The drumbeat of CANCER, CANCER, CANCER pounds away in the back of the head, insinuating itself into every waking moment and even invading our dreams, refusing to let us forget it for a single moment.

It's not just us, the people in the eye of the storm, who are caught up in a whirlwind of new, unfamiliar feelings and pressing practical needs. Sometimes those closest to the epicentre are so swept up in the turbulence of their own emotions, their own reactions, that they cannot be much help.

*My wife was just wonderful (up until my diagnosis, I thought I was the luckiest man in the world), but she was crap about cancer. She had this huge insecurity, this fear that I'd croak and leave her with four young children. She was so frightened but she couldn't admit it. Had she been honest about her feelings, it might have been different. But she found it difficult to ask for the support she needed. 'No,' she said, tight-lipped, to all offers of help, 'I'm fine.' But she wasn't. She was alone and frightened and burdened and she just couldn't cope. And when it was all over, she found it impossible to commit to the relationship. Looking back, it was the beginning of the end of the marriage.* Charlie Wilson

When those in the inner sanctum fall apart, friends who are on the periphery, and have the advantage of a little distance, can really come into their own.

*You feel the love of your friends and family in a way that you normally don't. An extraordinary number of people were there for me, including some quite surprising ones, people I hardly knew. They showed me how they felt in such a demonstrative way, I was stunned by the level of care and affection. To begin with I insisted*

23

*I was fine, I could cope. Then I let them in, and let them help, and it made the biggest difference.* Heidi Locher

## TAKE US AS YOU FIND US

People respond to the news that they have a life-threatening disease in all sorts of different, and often unpredictable, ways. The most panic-prone can become preternaturally calm, rising to the occasion in a way that can leave their friends stunned and even awestruck, while the steady, sensible types may temporarily whirl off-balance. Leave your preconceptions at home. Accept us as you find us, and as the people we always were: requiring no special pitying voices, no different treatment, no deep, meaningful looks and embraces. Continue to argue with us about politics and football. Hug us if you always have. Otherwise respect your distance.

Treat us as normally as you can and the odds are you'll soon find any distance and awkwardness dissolving. 'It was wonderful to see you, particularly as you are so much your old self,' emailed one friend a couple of months following my diagnosis, after we'd met up for lunch. 'Somehow I'd imagined you horribly altered, and so it was reassuring to see you still feisty and funny and full of life.'

*I knew someone with cancer and I treated them normally. They liked that because everyone else treated them like they were ill all the time.* Jade Goody

*Culturally, we tend to back off the possibility of death, and that can make the person who is facing this huge catastrophe in their lives feel very lonely, very isolated. The first thing is not to be afraid, to be able to see this person who you love and have had a long relationship with as the person they have always been. They may be facing something overwhelming and horrible, but their personality doesn't change. Their essence is the same. Keep that in mind and it becomes a bridge so that their illness isn't compounded by loneliness.* Tessa Jowell

*In an odd sort of way, I think one must let instinct take over. Go with the flow. It's about getting the balance right between 'Life goes on' and 'I'm here more than ever for you'. It's about offering without intruding. It's about milestones, fixing holidays together six months ahead, helping to build confidence and yet not suddenly coming up with grandiose plans that you would never have made if things had been 'normal'. Yet things ARE normal. We are still the friends, loved ones, neighbours we always were. It's just that we are a bit more conscious of it than we used to be.* Jon Snow

*The thing is, people are different with me now and I want them to be normal. After we first heard about my mum, people kept coming up to me at school and saying, 'How are you?' The teachers told the other girls I was having a hard time and then everyone came up to me, asking 'What's happened to your mum?' and nagging me to tell them: that was very annoying.* Clemmie Stebbings (aged 12)

25

Accept, too, that as we go through many different phases during the course of an illness that is itself unpredictable, how we feel at the moment may not be at all the same as how we will feel next Friday or in a fortnight or even 10 minutes from now.

*I have found that the best way to deal with a situation in which my emotional equanimity is as settled as the weather is to educate those friends who can hear with the following comments:*
*1. Not fine, bloody awful in fact, but I don't want to talk about it today, please call me tomorrow.*
*2. If you say poor thing to me one more time, I will hang up and never speak to you again.*
*3. Don't snivel round here, that's my line, get your own scriptwriter.*
*4. Not fine at all, I need a friend to cry on, can you come over RIGHT NOW?*
*5. It's OK to mention the word cancer in front of me, I promise not to throw up or pass out, life does in fact go on.* Sally Hamilton

## WHAT SORT OF FRIEND ARE YOU?
*We found we had two sorts of friends. There are the people who say rather helplessly 'I wish there was something I could do' and there are the people who stick a casserole on your doorstep or share a 25-mile round trip to the Royal Marsden in Sutton or throw their house open to you so you do not have to bear the long haul home every night. And you quickly discover that this is not really to do with how close they are to you as friends, but whether they*

26

*happen to be good at it or not. There are people who are good at dinner parties and people who are good on holidays, and then there are people who are good at compassion. They are the people who can empathise. Not sympathise. You don't need sympathy. What you need is someone who can put themselves in your place and see where the need is, who will listen while you endlessly bore on about platelets and blood counts without switching off or reaching for a newspaper or doodling on the back of an envelope.*
Maureen Lipman

*Since I was diagnosed with cancer last October, I have never (a) slept so badly, (b) spent so much time at the hairdresser and (c) been so popular. I am sick of being everyone's favourite cripple – you wouldn't believe the number of acquaintances who suddenly want to be your best friend and feel they are entitled to regular, blow-by-blow accounts of your emotional/psychological state. 'But Ruth, how ARE you?' they ask, meaningfully. Rubber-neckers.* Ruth Picardie, *Before I Say Goodbye*

## TAKE NO FOR AN ANSWER
Sometimes friends may genuinely not want our help. Their way of managing is by forging on regardless, requiring no special measures from anyone around them. Then, as this example shows, we help most by respecting this, by carrying on with life and business as normal, by recognising that 'The only way to help is not to help at all'.

27

*Cancer? Help! Until recently you could scarcely mention the Big C by name. Like the D\*\*\*l in a Victorian novel or the Evil One in Harry Potter, it was a dreadful visitation by malign forces beyond our ken, and usually beyond medical science. And only to be referred to in hushed tones. Well the science is better now, and I think we are all better talking about carcinomas, tumours, chemo and radiotherapy, and the rest of it. So just being there to talk about it might be the best help we can give.*

*Not always, though. I had a friend and colleague who was struck down, out of the blue, as I suppose you always are, by a brain tumour. He told us about it on a need-to-know basis. Reluctantly admitting that his time off work was caused by medical problems, and that his slurring of speech came not from a sudden predilection for afternoon drinking, he underwent a tricky operation from which he returned with a rakish eyepatch and a rather theatrical walking stick. After which he recovered completely, but only until his tumour returned a couple of years later. But from then on he was having no talk of his problems. The tumour may have been out to kill him, but in the meantime he was determined it wasn't going to ruin his life. And he certainly didn't want to talk about it. The only way to help was not to help at all. It was how he coped.* Clive Anderson

Offers of help can be like an answer to a prayer or they can be intrusive and unwanted. Bombarded by so many well-meant sincere offers, it can be difficult to say, 'Thanks very much, but no', especially when the offers are so well intentioned. If we find it hard to say 'No', a trusted friend who can say 'No' on our behalf is of infinite value. I gradually learnt that life really now was both too short and too precious to be polite for the sake of it, to have to endure calls or visits that I knew would be draining. Over time, I developed a self-preservational inner steeliness.

Good friends, true friends, also need to be able to hear a 'No' without taking offence, to intuit the difference between 'No, not at all' and 'Not for now, but maybe later', and to back off accordingly, accepting that, for example, this is not a good time to visit, without immediately pressing to fix another date.

*Some friends were overpowering. They meant well, but I felt battered by it. It was hard to summon the strength to thank them for their concern and to ask them to let me work things out in my own way.* Stanley Smith

*One of the luxuries of having cancer – and there aren't many – is the increased ruthlessness it allows you in dealing with people. If a bore or a sponger invites himself around to see you, you say no. If an invitation to a dull dinner party arrives, you turn it down. Conversely, if you need to see a real friend, then you ask for their company or invite yourself to their house, because there is no room for shyness any more.* Martyn Harris, 'This is not the time to die', *The Spectator*, 19 August 1995

*There were some people I wanted to see and others I didn't want around. There's a way of being sympathetic and supportive without saying 'Isn't it terrible?' all the time. People who were practical and sensitive to how I was feeling, who just knew how to put the cup of tea in the right place, were great, but others made demands on my time and my attention and my energy I just couldn't cope with. They meant well, but I learnt to get tougher. I would never have predicted that this illness would teach me not to be so polite.*
Dr Ann McPherson

*As the author's husband, the tidal wave of love and affection for Deborah and all of us was an enormous support. Don't, however, be surprised if not all kind invitations to lunch and a drink 'to talk about it' are taken up. Having broken the news to close friends and relatives, I soon learnt not to do a string of late evening calls, as these only became more and more downbeat, leaving both parties sunk in gloom. Instead, I would wait till an upbeat moment with the family – a boozy lunch with laughter – before bringing the next instalment of news. This way, those not immediately with her could be left with a positive conversation to dwell on before my next call. Remember, too, that all children react differently in these circumstances (for this reason, perhaps, our two older children later said they were grateful to have had the news broken to them individually, rather than as a group, which was how we had originally intended to do it), yet at the same time are trying to protect us, as parents, from their own fears for the future.* Charlie Stebbings

## STRIKE THE BALANCE BETWEEN SAD AND SOLEMN

In our new touchy-feely-weepy culture, there's a perception that crying together is very bonding and supportive, enabling a person to feel less lonely in their grief and shock and sorrow. All the people I talked to, however, found other people's tears and fears burdensome. 'It takes a degree of sheer physical will-power to endure not just the diagnosis and treatments, but the sympathy and sorrow of one's friends,' said one.

*Having people breaking down in tears or wanting/needing an emotional love-in was definitely NOT what I wanted. Even seeing tears well up in someone else's eyes used to turn me into a quivering jelly.* Rachel Williams

*I don't like people crying around me, especially if they are grown-ups, because then I think the situation is really bad. It makes me feel sad and I don't like it. Crying does not make me feel better. I know it is supposed to be good for you, but I don't like it.* Clemmie Stebbings (aged 12)

*Thinking back to when my mother was diagnosed with pancreatic cancer (which is bleak), I can of course remember a lot of people 'being marvellous'. But I can also remember a lot of people (albeit well-meaningly) 'being crap'. My father called them 'the ghouls', and they were the ones who sent cards with sunsets or soft-focus autumns saying, effectively, 'in deepest sympathy'. They were also the*

31

*ones who started talking to Mum in their special 'Death' voices.*

*I'm not going to say she only wanted people who could have a laugh about it, because she was always adamant that she wanted everyone to be devastated, but there is a difference between sad and solemn. I think I struck about the right balance in the first few weeks, but after that I got a bit bored and went back to tormenting her – my personal favourite being secretly activating her hospital bed so that the head and legs both lifted to put her in an amusing jack-knife position. The inflated surgical-glove-cum-udder, the cardboard potty as millinery, and gulping the patient's oxygen to alleviate hangovers, also passed the hours.*

*I even blow-dried her hair on the day before she died, which was frankly not the success I had hoped for, and which may – I now concede – have finished her off.* Hugh Grant

While there is no second-guessing what anyone will want and need from you (for some an embrace or hug can substitute for 1,000 words, while for others it can feel like a horrible infringement of personal space, especially when forced on them by those they don't know well), I found a surprising consensus about what people found helpful, or otherwise. Here is a summary:

**Helpful**
• 'A good friend sitting on my bed and just being there to lessen the loneliness, when trying to absorb the hugeness of what I'd just been told.'

32

• 'Beautiful flowers and plants that arrived in their own containers and didn't need decanting.'

• 'Uplifting letters with "No need to reply" at the bottom; gossipy emails ditto.'

• 'Having a friend on hand to answer the phone and tell well-wishers what was going on, especially boring ones.'

• 'Fielding people who called at the house and telling them when it was time to go.'

• 'People who treated whatever they did, however huge, as no big deal, the easiest thing in the world, rather than a grand gesture demanding my undying gratitude.'

**Unhelpful**

• 'People hanging round with long faces, feeling terrible and looking worse, and not knowing what to say or where to put themselves.'

• 'Having to feed well-wishers and make endless cups of tea.'

• 'Treating me like a hero/heroine.'

• 'Making assumptions about how I was feeling.'

33

- 'Being bombarded with questions and/or advice.'

- 'Arriving on the doorstep unannounced.'

- 'People who seemed to be enjoying the drama, or who were clearly using the situation as another piece of gossip.'

- 'Having to submit to intrusive questions and close embraces from people I hardly knew.'

- 'People who broke down and cried, leaving me to comfort them.'

# 1. *Hang back*

Unless you are a close friend, or one of the immediate family, or you know the person is comparatively unsupported and needs all the help they can get, do *not* rush round uninvited unless it is to leave a gift or plate of food at the door, with a note saying no reply needed. Chances are that telephone calls or requests for visits, though generously meant, will feel intrusive, and may even be interpreted as an attempt to meet for the final time. This is not the last-chance saloon. There will be time. So bide it.

Unless the diagnosis was expected, your friend is almost

certainly in shock. This is likely to be the worst thing that has ever happened to them. Allow them time to adapt to this often frightening turn of events, while you read through the suggestions in this book and see what you are best equipped to offer.

Do not take offence if offers of help and visits are met by a 'No' or you do not get an answer. Dozens or even hundreds of cards and letters may arrive following a diagnosis, along with so many phone calls, that it is impossible to reply to all of them. If you do not hear, don't be deterred. Wait a while and then ring a close friend or relative and try to establish when you might visit and/or where you might be able to help.

*My appetite vanished utterly, but chocolate brownies and shepherd's pies were very popular with everyone else.* Dee Dee Hope

# 2. *For the first contact, email or text rather than telephone, or send a card or letter*

All the above methods have the advantage of allowing recipients to reply when and as and if it suits them, and are therefore much less intrusive than telephoning or calling round in person.

When writing, there is no 'right response'. What's clear is that it's always better to make some overture, rather than to stay away or, as it may seem to the person involved, 'run a mile'. 'When I became ill,' reminisced one woman bitterly, 'people I had given hours of time to through their various crises simply vanished.'

Some sentiments are likely to be better received than others, but much depends upon the person. If you don't know what to write, say exactly that. Writing about how much you value your friendship, and adding some funny observations or reminiscences, will probably go down better than wading in with advice or half-baked theories as to causation.

I soon tired of all that rallying stuff about 'You're such a fighter, I'm sure you can beat it' or 'Knowing you, your strong spirit will prevail and you will never give up that battle'. I know they meant well, but these warlike sentiments made me feel that if I didn't respond to treatment it could count as 'giving up', as though I hadn't tried – or rather fought – hard enough and I was somehow letting the side down. I found those stories of people my friends had known personally who, despite the few short months or weeks they had been 'given', were still in their gardens planting bulbs and pruning the roses, much more cheering.

*I'm a great believer in letters. It's often easier to write things than to say them, and more likely that you will finish what you want to say.* Tessa Jowell

*After the initial shock of finding out that Mum had cancer, all I wanted to do was lock up that part of my life in a tiny box that*

36

*only needed to be opened when really necessary. But it can't work like that when the phone is going every three minutes with people wondering how your mum is and her having to tell and retell her story. Emails were definitely the way forward.* Romilly Stebbings (aged 15)

**MOST IMPORTANT** Be sure to write that you don't expect a reply. The strain of feeling that one should be acknowledging letters and cards, takes away from the pleasure of receiving them. A PS at the end of a letter saying 'No need to reply' is a a present in itself.

*When you write, be sure to use the present tense.* One friend of mine was unnerved to receive a letter that went on for page after page, extravagantly praising all her qualities and achievements, but which was penned in the past tense. It was like reading her own obituary, she said.

# 3. *Volunteer your secretarial services*

The burden of thanking can be seriously daunting – 'like Christmas times 100', as one person put it. If your friend feels overwhelmed, a standard email can be sent out, thanking for thoughts and prayers and expressions of concern, and giving a few brief details.

You might also offer to respond to letters and cards, and

thank for gifts, on your friend's behalf. Ask him or her to dictate a couple of paragraphs that you can use for everyone, and then type it into a word document on the computer; date and print off as necessary, and your friend can then add a closing personal sentence. Address and stamp all the envelopes and take them to the post.

> **NB** If the emails are coming thick and fast, you can either compose an auto reply (look on menu options in the toolbar or enter 'auto reply' in your email programme's help box), which can be sent automatically to anyone in the address book, or you can compose a standard message, leaving the address blank, and click 'save as draft', adding email addresses and sending out as necessary.

## 4. *Offer to be a conduit of information*

Breaking the news can be a huge emotional burden. On top of your friend's own grief and fear comes the task of comforting and reassuring all those who love them. Would it help if you took down a list of those people who needn't hear it first-hand and who you can ring with the news? Be sure to listen to instructions about how much (or little) contact will be welcome (not everyone is allergic to the doorbell and/or telephone), and how much medical information should be disseminated. Some people are very open. Others are averse to having all but the most basic details of their condition broadcast. And may even swear you to secrecy.

*When my sister was diagnosed with cancer, she couldn't cope, didn't want to see anyone and withdrew completely. But the word soon got out, so I took on the role of answering the phone and trying to deal with people wanting to come round. She'd generally stay upstairs, while I invited them in, made them tea, thanked them for their concern, filled them in, made them feel included, put their flowers in water and sent them on their way.* Pamela Barry

## 5. *Be a clinic companion*

It is now accepted that many people will want to bring a friend or relative to the endless clinics, scans and consultations that follow in the wake of a cancer diagnosis (I remember being gobsmacked at how many people I was lined up to see within the first five days). Someone at one remove from the shock and horror is in a better position to remember what is said ('The serious information slithered around in my brain like mercury, ungraspable,' wrote Kate Carr in *It's Not Like That, Actually*), to ask the doctors to clarify what they are saying (and, if necessary, to translate medicalese into plain English) and, after the consultation is over, to offer another view of what was said.

As a companion, you can also do much to alleviate the tedium of waiting, if only by chatting or doing the crossword together, or fetching tea or coffee. I found it particularly spoiling to be picked up and dropped at the appointment by car or taxi, while my companion bothered with parking and paying.

*I always loved it when friends drove me to the hospital and waited with me while I went for appointments and treated it as no big deal, just ordinary.* Julia Darling

Most valuable, however, were those friends who made it their business to be truly on the ball; who would take a notebook and pencil, asking me what questions I wanted answers to, asterisking the three or four most urgent ones, so they could prompt me if, as was likely, I forgot some of them.

**DID YOU KNOW?** Studies show that patients recall only a quarter of what is said to them in medical consultations and that this figure can drop to just one-tenth if they are under severe stress.

You might like to consider taking a tape recorder and asking whether you can record the consultation. A few specialists are now starting to make tapes as a matter of course, handing them over to patients as they leave. It means they can replay the consultation when they are in a better position to absorb the information, and can also play it to close family so that they know what has been discussed.

*My youngest son advised me to take a tape recorder to all my examinations and clinic appointments. I found this invaluable as I tended to become confused and would forget what the doctor had said, hesitating to ask again for fear of being thought a complete nitwit. During the month, I would write down in my diary everything that bothered me, and every question that I wanted answered on the day of my next appointment, and armed with this and my tape recorder, I felt relaxed at my consultations. I would play my tape two, three and even four times over when I returned home, ensuring that I missed nothing.* Hannah Lurie

**Remind your friend that he or she can:**

• Put as many questions to the doctors as needed about the proposed treatment, and its side-effects, in order to make informed decisions. Don't be put off by a general air of busyness – the impression that some doctors have raised to an art form that their time is just too valuable to go through things in detail. Ask them to explain – and in words your friend can understand.

• Take time before making any decisions regarding treatment. Many people's abiding memory of their diagnosis is the terrifying speed with which they were swept on to the cancer conveyor belt, leaving no time for calm consideration or a second opinion. 'It's not a medical emergency,' says Dr John Toy, medical director of Cancer Research UK, who advises taking as much time as one needs thinking through one's treatment options. 'You haven't been knocked down in the street, though you may feel like you have. Decisions can always wait at least a few days.'

• Ask to be referred to an oncologist (cancer expert) or a surgeon with specific expertise if the cancer is rare or is one in which the doctor has relatively little experience.

• Request to see their medical records (a recognised 'right' since 1991, though doctors can occasionally refuse access if they believe such information could be harmful) and to have all letters copied to them.

• Ask for a second opinion if they are unhappy about their doctor's view.

• Talk to their GP if they are unhappy with any aspect of their care.

• Change to another GP if, after talking to their current doctor, they continue to be unhappy with the way they are being treated.

• Make a complaint – directly or via Pals (Patient Advice and Liaison Services) or via a third party. Download the Patients Association's excellent online publication *How to Make a Complaint* (at www.patients-association.com), or ring the helpline (0845 608 4455, Monday to Friday, 10am to 4pm).

**IMPORTANT** Before leaving, ask if there is someone your friend can ring if further questions arise, and note down a contact name and number. Those with the commoner cancers (breast, bowel, lung, prostate) should be offered a clinical nurse specialist. This key person is not just a friendly face in the clinic, but someone patients can rely on to give advice and support on a whole range of issues, from what grants and entitlements they might be eligible for to getting travel insurance when going away on holiday.

**TIP** If your friend has quite a list of questions, and needs more time than usual to talk, try to secure the last appointment of the day. From my experience, this is usually the least sought-after slot because it generally entails more waiting. Yet, once all the other patients on the list have been seen, I have found my oncologist more relaxed about letting time run on while he answers all my questions and, very often, by so doing puts my mind at rest.

# 6. *Offer to check that the treatment being offered is the gold standard for the type and stage of cancer*

Having cancer brings so many unsettling uncertainties, it can be a big relief to know that the therapy being proposed is the same as would be given by any of the country's top teaching hospitals or centres of excellence. The National Institute for Clinical Excellence (NICE) publishes detailed national standards of care for people with specific types of cancer in England and Wales, called *Improving Outcomes.* Visit www.nice.org.uk (click on 'Want to read our guidance on an illness or condition?', click on 'Cancer' and then on the particular type). A similar guide to standards of care is produced by NHS Quality Improvement Scotland; you can find it at www.nhshealthquality.org.

Although reliable, independent, up-to-date information on all local hospitals is not yet widely available, you may also be able to find out how the hospital in question is performing on reducing waiting times for treatment and on prescribing Nice-recommended cancer drugs, and even survival rates, so giving your friend the choice to stay put or request referral to a better hospital further afield.

# 7. *Become an information-gatherer*

The old adage 'Information is power' couldn't be more true, as long as the information is well balanced and accurate. There is even some research to show that well-informed, inquiring patients tend to do better than those who do not ask and accept whatever they are given, probably because the former stick their necks out and demand certain treatments, right down to being prepared to move hospital when these are not available.

However assertive a person normally is, it's not easy to be a dynamic, questing, 'take charge' sort of patient when whacked by something as potentially serious as a diagnosis of cancer, especially if, as in my case, it comes with the specific advice not to embark on an internet search, 'as you'll only terrify yourself'. Though a health journalist myself, and not naturally one to bury my head in the sand, I had enough self-knowledge to realise that my consultant had a point: I was so saturated with bad news, I couldn't deal with one more single gloomy survival statistic or poor response rate. I needed someone to sift the good from the bad, identify the promising and protect me from the depressing.

Fortunately, a friend, Olivia Timbs, a well-respected medical journalist and editor of *The Pharmaceutical Journal*, generously volunteered to do the job for me. She retrieved a mass of information and scientific papers, and sent it to me in concise, digestible form via a series of emails, sparing me precious time and, just as important, the need to confront some unpalatable statistics along the way.

If your friend, like me, is an ostrich (even if only a temporary one), but loath to miss out on any new treatments that might be available, and you are medically trained and/or technologically literate, you, too, can oh-so-usefully sift through the statistics, extracting useful information and passing it on in bite-sized chunks.

*Because I've had a chronic kidney condition since I was a child, medical terminology doesn't frighten me and hospitals are like a second home for me. But when Nazira found out she had breast cancer, it was a new experience for her – filled with fear and anxiety. She was also overcome by the information being thrown at her. So I went on the internet, did a lot of research, read the medical journals and found out a lot of information. Being scientifically minded with a degree in electronics, I could understand the language and make sense of the statistics. And then we'd sit down and chat, and I'd ask her what she wanted to do. How did she feel? What if this happened, or that? Rather than bombarding her with information, I gave it to her a little bit at a time in a way that made sense to her. She trusted me completely. We became a team.*
Shoky Visram

*It's extremely difficult to take in bad news. Cancer, even if it is*

46

*treatable, is such bad news that the first reaction is to go into shock; the brain feels numb, and it's impossible to frame questions, to sort out plans, to ask what the next steps are. So phoning a friend can give everyone the opportunity to work out exactly what questions to ask the healthcare professionals about treatment and prognosis, and the available support; all the information that seems so obvious when it's not happening to you, but so confusing when it is.* Esther Rantzen

With a child, where the sense of helplessness is total, making it your role to be informed on their behalf can be as therapeutic for the parent (or aunt or grandparent or godparent or close friend) as for the child.

*It's very humbling to watch a child fighting for her life. When she was very ill and close to death, as she was three times, it felt like it was Georgie and me battling away together. She regarded me as her guardian angel. I'd sit at the end of her bed and quiz the doctors endlessly. She knew that I had made it my business to know everything I needed to know. She knew and believed we were doing all we could, that the doctors were doing all they could.* Nicola Horlick

Never make assumptions about what a person with a new diagnosis will, or won't, want to know. In my experience, the ostrich tendency is really quite common, even among doctors.

*I call them the information mafia. One of my colleagues insisted on ringing me and telling me what my survival chances were for my type and stage of breast cancer when actually I really didn't want to know at that moment – though I recognise he was only trying to be helpful.* Dr Ann McPherson

As life settles down again, your friend may want to resume control, recognising that information and knowledge can be a lifeline out of helplessness and fear, that terrifying feeling of being the victim. 'The more I know, the more secure I feel,' says a friend who has stomach cancer. 'Even if the news is bad, knowledge soothes me. The worst part is not knowing, not being told, that niggling feeling that someone somewhere knows something that I don't.'

*Caroline wanted to be free to handle her illness in her own way. It gave her strength. She was a teacher and took this academic, scholarly approach to her cancer. My son got her going on the internet, and she'd sit at the computer and do her research and then turn up at the hospital with some paper she had found from the University of Texas Medical School. I think she thoroughly frightened her consultant, who couldn't possibly keep up with it, but it helped her enormously to feel she was retaining some control.* Tony Benn

*When I was found to have a non-invasive breast tumour, called a*

*ductal carcinoma in situ, back in 1984, the doctors kept trying to tell me it wasn't breast cancer because they thought I couldn't take it. But they couldn't have been more wrong. I'd rather face anything head-on, however horrible. From my point of view, the very worst thing is not being told enough, not being able to get the information. I can deal with almost anything if I know what it is. Over the years, I've acted as an information-gatherer for several friends, particularly one who had a very rare form of ovarian cancer that the doctors over here didn't have much expertise in. I managed to put her in touch with a specialist team in Boston, and she went to the US for her treatment. That was 13 years ago, and she's doing very well.* Rabbi Julia Neuberger

**IMPORTANT** CancerBACUP produces a series of information booklets on all but the rarest cancers, which can be either downloaded off the internet (www.cancerbacup.org.uk) or sent on request, free of charge (call 0808 800 1234, Monday to Friday, 9am to 7pm). America's National Cancer Institute (www.nci.nih.gov) also has comprehensive information on all cancer types, along with the low-down on any new cancer treatments: enter 'newly approved cancer treatments' in the search box and it will take you to an alphabetical listing. *The British Journal of Cancer* (www.nature.com/bjc) reports regularly on recent trial results and gives perspectives on new drugs, as does *The Pharmaceutical Journal* (www.pharmj.com; use the search facility). Journals usually charge for the full text of any paper, but the short summary, or abstract, often gives sufficient detail. Maggie's Centres (www.maggiescentres.org) provides a long list of useful websites that have been vetted for content (click on 'Resources', then 'Cancer Information', then on one of four various links). Subscribe to *The British Medical Journal*'s free daily round-up of medical news stories and also ask for email alerts to be posted whenever features on the relevant cancer appear (www.bmj.com; click on 'Email alerts' under 'Services' in the left-hand toolbar).

# 8. *Find out about clinical trials*

The cancer experts I have spoken to over the years say almost as one that they would move heaven and earth to get themselves on to a clinical trial. Because of the strict procedural guidelines that govern any trial, the standard of care is generally extremely high, which probably explains why research shows that, regardless of whether or not they receive the active treatment, patients who are registered within a trial tend to do better than a comparative group of patients who are not.

**NB** It is important to check what clinical trials may be taking place *before* treatment begins, as previous therapy can often make a person ineligible. The CancerBACUP website (www.cancerbacup.org.uk) has a list of all ongoing trials in the

UK, with details of who is running them and how to make contact. You can help friends by searching for trials that are currently recruiting patients with their type of cancer and, especially, checking the eligibility criteria so that they do not go ahead and embark on treatment that might then disqualify them from these trials (click on 'Trials', 'Cancer type' and 'All'). With so many ongoing clinical trials (92 different breast cancer treatments alone at the last count), it's always helpful to print out details of those that might be appropriate and to ask the consultant about them.

## 9. *Find out who to contact for a second opinion*

Time was when to request a second opinion might have been considered a vote of no confidence in one's doctor; now, with several treatment options often under discussion and the possibility of enrolling in clinical trials of new drugs and/or treatments, it is looked on as a perfectly sensible move. I have had at least three 'second' opinions. My wonderfully patient oncologist is happy to indulge my quest for knowledge and comparative information, as long as I am completely open about it. I try to phrase each request as tactfully as I can, telling him who I would like to consult and when, and even though it means extra work for him writing letters and organising for my notes to be photocopied or faxed (in one case, through to the US), he has yet to take offence. Quite understandably, doctors, like any professionals, tend to get upset when second opinions are sought behind their backs.

Once your friend has a name (or you have found one), ask the oncologist to write a referral letter. If finances permit, it may be worth considering paying for this consultation privately so as not to delay the start of any treatment that has been proposed.

*I was unhappy with the attitude of my first surgeon, but didn't want to offend him and, in my shock at all that was going on, was too wishy-washy to look for anyone else. And I'm a health professional! So my sister-in-law phoned Edinburgh and got chatting to a breast specialist on my behalf, and I ended up with the loveliest surgeon in the world who I had absolute trust in.* Vicky Baglioni

## 10. *Find out if your friend can be put in touch with a Macmillan nurse*

All Macmillan nurses are clinical nurse specialists in palliative care with at least two years of experience in the field. They work in hospitals, the community and hospices, and currently number around 2,500. Along with palliative care, Macmillan nurses use their specialist skills to provide emotional support, effective pain relief, liaison with other nursing services, advice on symptom control, and information on anything that might arise in the wake of cancer diagnosis and treatment.

NHS palliative care nurses working in the community fulfil much the same role. I certainly took fright when I was told soon after my diagnosis that I was going to be contacted by a palliative care nurse. I thought that this happens only to people right at the end of their lives, and I had no intention of being prematurely consigned to my coffin. But from the moment Maggie Bisset arrived at my door, I recognised that she was there to make my life easier in whatever way she could.

She advised me, she organised prescriptions for my pain relief, she was endlessly reassuring about the symptoms that were keeping me awake at night. She guided me through the maze of different services on offer and helped me to claim the benefits I was entitled to but which I, like so many others, knew nothing about. She arranged a Home Office licence that allowed me to take morphine out of the country, and put me in touch with travel insurers. There was nothing Maggie wouldn't take on. After 10 years of working with seriously ill people, and their families, nothing surprised or shocked her.

Soon after we had broken the news to our four children, she arrived on the doorstep like an answer to a prayer and talked to them while I made myself scarce upstairs, so that they could ask any questions that were preying on their minds, and could voice the fears that they didn't feel they could, or should, talk about in front of my husband and myself.

**HOW TO FIND A MACMILLAN/PALLIATIVE CARE NURSE** Macmillan nurses can provide help and support at any time after someone has been diagnosed with cancer. Usually, the consultant, GP, district nurse or clinical nurse specialist will make a referral, using locally agreed guidelines (not all areas of the country are covered), at the request of the individual, a close friend or family member. There is no charge for a Macmillan/palliative care nurse.

# 11. *Offer to put your friend in touch with a support group/someone with a similar type of cancer or who has had the treatment being proposed*

There's a level of connection, if not identification, among people who have, or have had, cancer that even one's closest and most warm-hearted friends can never match. I now have a circle of new friends – originally friends of friends – who date from AD (After the Diagnosis). With each other, we can voice hopes too fragile, fears too dark and jokes too black to be shared with anyone else, along with the nitty-gritty of everyday cancer care: from the details of a particular medicated mouthwash to guard against mouth ulcers during chemo to names of the more palatable brands of green tea (there aren't many).

Would your friend be interested in talking to 'a friendly stranger' (see Corin Redgrave's contribution over the page)? Namely, someone with the same sort of cancer, who may have experienced the treatment that your friend will be undergoing? Alternatively, you could try introducing them to a whole new band of virtual friends via a website such as the award-winning DIPEx (www.dipex.org; click 'Experiences' in the top toolbar), which has videotaped stories of people with the seven most common cancers and runs an interactive forum for sharing experiences and thoughts. The site, which averages almost a million hits a month, was co-founded by the Oxford GP Ann McPherson after her own experience of breast cancer left her aware that, while she was well genned up medically, talking to others with the same problem about what it was really like to have the disease gave her a different sort of information. 'I'm quite well in with all this stuff, I'm married to a breast cancer epidemiologist, so I didn't need straight facts. It was more that I learnt so much from other patients, and we tried to capture that when we set up the website.'

Or try the real thing: there are now more than 700 local support groups around the UK run on a voluntary basis by people who have experience of cancer, either directly or through a family member or friend. Talking to others who have had similar experiences can help people feel less frightened and isolated, and may also help to show them that there is a way through these feelings, and the proposed treatment, and out the other side. Macmillan Cancer Relief publishes a directory of cancer support groups (contact the Macmillan CancerLine on 0808 808 2020).

If your friend is geographically lucky enough to live near one of the five Maggie's Centres that are up and running (in Edinburgh, Glasgow, Dundee, Inverness and Oxford), or the further six under development (in Fife, Lanarkshire, London, Nottingham, Cheltenham and Cambridge), give them the details (www.maggiescentres.org).

These centres were the brainchild of Maggie Keswick Jencks. After hearing a piece of particularly devastating news about the spread of her own cancer, she was sitting trying to absorb the enormity of it when she was asked if she could please vacate the chair she was sitting on as another patient would be needing it. At that moment, she determined to set up a series of non-institutional centres attached to major NHS hospitals, where there would always be plenty of seats for everyone; where people could take all the time they needed to adjust to their diagnosis; and where they could access support that would enable them to be as healthy in mind and body as possible, and make their own contribution to their medical treatment and recovery.

*The bush telegraph was just fantastic: the best thing doctors and friends did for me was to put me in touch with other men who had had prostate cancer and had undergone the various treatments I was now considering. These ex-patients were, without exception, wonderfully generous with their time and their advice. One man, who used to be the chief paramedic of the London Ambulance Service, has since become quite a good friend. We still correspond and he comes to see my shows.*

*What you need is a friendly stranger: someone with whom you can share the most intimate details and who will be absolutely unfazed by your questions about what lies ahead. They will also tell you things that the surgeons don't: that cranberry juice is very good post-operatively for internal bleeding, for example, or that cups of coffee are 100 per cent guaranteed to upset the stomach.* Corin Redgrave

*In the village where we live, the five or six people who have or have had cancer call themselves the BBC – the Beat the Bugger Club – and meet for supper or drinks about once a month to exchange information about what is available locally in terms of treatment and resources, and to support newcomers who have been diagnosed. Each of them swears by it.* Andro Linklater

*I began to remember the odd friend who had been through chemo (I didn't know many) and bravely rang them up. 'How was it for you?' I asked. Just to talk to people who had been through it was energising.* Mary MacCarthy

*There's nothing like meeting people who have had your cancer, and*

*gone through it, and are not only still alive but abundantly, evidently well. When a friend developed breast cancer recently, I took her to Breast Cancer Care's fashion show, not so much for the clothes or the occasion, though they were fun, but because I knew that meeting volunteers who had been living with the disease for years and years and years would boost her spirits more than I ever could.* Cherie Blair, patron of Breast Cancer Care

Be prepared for a 'No'. While some people find it enormously helpful and reassuring to talk to people undergoing similar experiences, others shrink from any such contact and most emphatically do *not* want to 'join the club'.

*I found any association with the hospital scary, and I still have difficulty talking to people who have had or who are going through the same ordeal. Reliving memories leaves me feeling wobbly, and a little frightened when I am reminded of the potential seriousness of my situation.* Georgie Hall

*I hated attending the chemotherapy suite. The waiting, the smells, the patients with their gallows humour. I dreaded some diseased old bloke asking me what I was in for and getting a blow-by-blow account of his colostomy while he asked me probing questions about the size, stage and grade of the tumour so recently excised from my breast. I felt too young to be there and I was determined to be absolutely not like them with their cheery cracks and 'mustn't*

*grumble' optimism. I wasn't in their 'club' and definitely
wasn't signing up to their banter about 'neutrophil counts' and
'chemo-fevers'. So I sat with a book and pretended none of it was
happening.* Clare Stanley

> **NB** Macmillan CancerLine advisers are also there to listen, to
> offer information and emotional support by phone, letter and
> email, and can give contact details of specific organisations
> that may be able to put your friend in touch with some-
> one with a similar type of cancer (0808 808 2020 or
> cancerline@macmillan.org.uk).

# 12. *Stoke hope*

However grim our prognoses, we all need to feel that we will be
in the exceptional few per cent who make it past a year, or five
years or even 10. Call it denial if you will, but those of us living with cancer (especially cancer that has metastasised to those
so-called no-hope sites of lungs, liver, bones and brain) find
such hope sustaining.

Not long after my own diagnosis, a friend sent me an
email giving me the web-link to *The Median Isn't the Message*
(www.cancerguide. org/median_not_msg.html), a marvellous
essay by the evolutionary biologist Stephen Jay Gould, who was
diagnosed with abdominal mesothelioma, an incurable cancer,

at the age of 40. He found out that it carried a median mortality rate of just eight months after diagnosis.

Faced with such a statistic, most people would conclude that this meant they had about that long to live – plus a couple of months if they were lucky. But Gould, who was good at maths, worked out that there must be a very long tail on the far side of the median composed of those people who lived for much longer, and he worked out that he had a good chance of being one of them. He was right, and he lived for another 20 years, finishing his life's work, *The Structure of Evolutionary Theory*, in the process.

Stories of these 'statistical outliers', the people who beat the odds, confound their doctor's expectations and generally make nonsense of the statistics, are inspiring. Just one such is the Olympic cyclist Lance Armstrong, who was diagnosed with stage IV testicular cancer in 1996, with tumours in his lung and brain, but recovered after treatment to win the Tour de France in 1999 and virtually every year since. The less spectacular reality is that millions of cancer patients *do* go on to make full recoveries, a fact that often fails to reach the headlines.

*The balance doesn't seem to be there. I know so many people who have had cancer and who are in their 10th or 15th or 20th year. I can count at least 10. And yet there's such a fear we only remember the people who died, we only hold on to the statistics of the negative.* Felicity Kendal

*Even when her consultants were saying, 'It's a miracle she's still standing up', because there were quite a few tumours on her spine, Caron was convinced she was going to beat it, and so were we. She'd outlived all the predictions. Underneath the surface I was worried sick, but she never gave up hope and she was right. Miracles do happen, situations change and drugs are improving all the time.* Gloria Hunniford

**NB** New research from the Royal Marsden Hospital, which tracked 500 women for 10 years, found that women who were classed as having a 'helpless' or 'hopeless' response to their diagnosis were at greater risk of relapse and early death. The authors do not explain why a hopeful outlook should have an effect on disease-free survival, though various possible mechanisms have been suggested, including an effect on the immune system. Nevertheless, the authors state: 'Having found evidence of an adverse impact on disease-free survival of a hopeless/helpless response at 10 years post-diagnosis, the aim now would be to clarify the mechanisms of action and develop suitable therapies in order to help improve outcomes in these women.' *European Journal of Cancer*, April 2005

*Hope does not arise from being told to 'think positively', or from hearing an overly rosy forecast. Hope is rooted in unalloyed reality. Hope is the elevating feeling we experience when we see – in the mind's eye – a path to a better future. Hope acknowledges the*

61

*significant obstacles and deep pitfalls along that path. True hope has no room for delusion, but gives us the courage to confront our circumstances and the capacity to surmount them... For all my patients, hope, true hope, has proved as important as any medication I might prescribe or any procedure I might perform.*
Dr Jerome Groopman, *The Anatomy of Hope*

## 13. *Be a breath of fresh air*

Cancer quickly comes to dominate one's life to the point where it becomes quite a challenge to fit in anything else between the hospital visits and clinic appointments and visits to complementary practitioners. Friends who offer cancer vacations, mini-breaks that take us out of ourselves and our situation, are worth their weight in gold – giving us something to look forward to in a future that may otherwise be filled with dread.

*When, at the age of 26, our daughter Anna was found to have not just cancer, but one of the rarest cancers known to man, she said I want quality of time, quality of life, no pity, no heads on one side saying 'poor Anna', and whenever possible, through the treatment, we are going to party. And party we did. She had 16 major operations in five years, but in between she'd set her sights on the next Robbie Williams or Barbra Streisand concert, or the next football match. She was a huge Arsenal fan. She would plot a shopping expedition or, memorably – and this was just weeks before she died – a This is Your Life programme about me, with her mother and the BBC. Having something to look forward to would give her this huge adrenalin rush. She'd get so excited, her spirits would lift and the symptoms would go out of the window, including the pain. As a family, we had some of the best times we'd ever had in those five years. And by the time she died, six days before her 32nd birthday, there was nothing left unsaid and nothing left undone.* Bob Wilson

Inspiration, laughter, poetry, music, something new and surprising that re-cements the friendship, helps to remove that perpetual dark cloud hanging on the horizon and reminds us of who we were before all this horribleness descended. 'My illness gradually took up so much of my time that I could no longer keep it in what I thought of as its place, control it,' wrote one person, speaking for many. 'I felt myself becoming my illness, the sum of my symptoms.'

*We were able to help three friends who suffered from cancer: my wife by giving regular lessons in the Alexander Technique, and I by continuing to treat them as the people I knew them to be and especially by encouraging them to listen to music in the concert hall.*

*If you sit at home listening to music, it locks you in on yourself, but go into the concert hall where there is all this unlikely activity, this blowing and scraping, and you have a chance of being lifted out of yourself, and your isolation can melt away. Great music is very healing. We know that children and cattle do better when you play Mozart. If you're listening to a composer like Mozart, it is so perfectly done, so obviously grounded in natural harmonics, it seems quite probable that it has a harmonising effect on the whole nervous system. He has always been an ever-present help in times of trouble to me.* Sir Colin Davis

*Life is doom-laden enough when you have cancer and I needed lightening up. Big time. Trivia made me feel normal.* Kate Carr, *It's Not Like That, Actually*

*Every week a friend would cut out things from the newspapers and magazines that she thought I might like or that would make me laugh and bundle them into an envelope. They took me right out of myself and never failed to lift my spirits. She was brilliant at finding funny cards, too.* Dee Dee Hope

*GOOD THINGS… Picking me up and taking me somewhere beautiful, like to see bluebells, then taking me home without mentioning illness; laughing with me; sending me a sachet of aphrodisiac tea (got one this morning); making compilation CDs of music I might like; talking about adventures, nature, food, anything. Illness gets so boring.* Julia Darling

# 14. *Offer the gift of a life experience they would not otherwise have had*

It doesn't have to be a *Jim'll Fix It* extravaganza. Some of the simplest gestures go down the best. Examples might range from a picnic in the garden with a group of old schoolfriends not glimpsed for decades, to a trip down memory lane to a childhood home, to tickets to a poetry reading or a Cup Final.

Whatever it is, don't just talk about it. If you get a positive response, do it. 'I felt appreciation whenever I took action, rather than just made plans,' reminisces Fran Bentley, who has had four good friends and a brother with cancer and is among my best half-dozen pin-up cancer pals. 'Many make promises lightly, but few carry them through.'

*When I took my great friend Sandy to India, she had recently had surgery for a brain tumour. Her prognosis was poor and there were some risks involved with air travel, but both of us wanted to take the opportunity to visit somewhere she had never been while it was still possible. I sought permission to take the risk directly from her partner and her parents so that, if the worst happened, the trip had their blessing. I shared the cost with another friend so there would be no financial burden on her.*

*Afterwards, Sandy wrote in a letter I treasure: 'How can I thank you enough for being so kind, generous and, indeed, brave to take me on such an adventure? My head is full of Goan green, with vivid orange flashes – indeed, all colours, textures, tastes, sounds – to keep flat grey February at bay. What a fantastic time we had!'*

*Best of all, she followed it up with a holiday of her own to the same place with her partner and children two months later. It was their first ever family holiday abroad, and I feel proud that I helped to give her the confidence to make it happen.* Frances Bentley

*When I was in the middle of having radiotherapy for my breast cancer, and had taken time off work, an epidemiologist friend of my husband, who is an expert on wild orchids, would take me to coppices and woods and meadows around Oxford, thanks to a local wildlife trust, and we'd have a bit of a treasure hunt. It was late spring and some of those rare and exotic blooms were quite disgusting-looking, albeit very unusual. One time we went into this field and it was full of pink and purple orchids and wild flowers. It was the beginning of June and just glorious, and I realised that here was something that I would never normally have had the chance or the time to do.* Dr Ann McPherson

*I'm doing something I really love to do – fused-glass art work – something I can't wait to get back to, something I dream about. Something totally new that doesn't come to me from my past, from anything anybody encouraged me to do. A real break with the past.* Treya Killam Wilber, *Grace and Grit*

# 15. *Maximise your laughs*

Does your friend really need to keep abreast of all the terrible
things that are happening in the world? One friend advised a
'news fast' as a way of insulating myself from the depressed state
of the world; another sent me the complete series of *The Vicar
of Dibley* on DVD, which never fails to raise a guffaw; yet
another friend sends funny, newsy, perfectly pitched letters that
always give me a lift.

*As we settled into a rhythm of fairly regular visiting, I started to see
that my role was to try to keep him laughing. John and I both
shared a wacky sense of humour about journalism and the world
around us, and I saw it as my job to make sure no matter how
much pain he was in, no matter how weak he was, we would have
at least one mild hysteria session every visit.* Alastair Campbell

*When a great friend, the actor Simon Cadell, had cancer, it was so
advanced it was in every cell in his body. We were told he had a
month to live, so we all wrote him letters and sent jokes, because he
had a great sense of humour. I told him a funny one I'd just heard
about a mutual actress friend in New York, and said, 'You can't go
without knowing this...' And another friend wrote, 'I fully expect
to see you in a voice-over studio in a year's time looking embarrassed.' Simon was king of the voice-overs and I thought it was a
very good way of dealing with it, of going beyond the predictable*

*'I'm so sorry'. Laughter is the best medicine. It is. And what's more, this friend turned out to be quite right. Simon went on to live for three more years. And good years, too.* Patricia Hodge

*You have to laugh. A friend and I went looking for wigs. You can get one on the NHS, you know. So we went to this place and it could have been so grim, but we had a hilarious time. I said, 'I want an Elvis wig', and this stiff little man said, 'We don't do novelty wigs. We match it as closely as we can to your own hair.' It was just so funny. So I got this wig, but I never wore it. The children used it for dressing up and thought it was great.* Charlie Wilson

*There was nothing my husband Richard wouldn't make fun of, nothing too sacred, nothing off-limits, nothing that couldn't be laughed at. It sounds black, but he'd call me the old sicko and say things like, 'We're going to do such and such on Friday', and I'd say, 'That sounds fun, count me in', and he'd say, 'Why? You won't be around by then.' Somehow not just looking at the monsters under the bed, but screeching with laughter at them, was a brilliant antidote to all the horror and the fear.* Heidi Locher

# What should
I say?

You may think that we live in a more open society, where everything and anything is up for discussion? Think again. The conversational strictures around cancer remain every bit as constraining as the Victorian embargo on sex. Forget b*****, 'cancer' is *definitely* the worst six-letter word in the language.

It's 'a long illness' in the 'Deaths' column of the newspaper, 'a blockage' or 'a little lump' in family stories about what happened to Auntie Gladys.

*I've lost count of the relatives who have met me at the door and said, 'Don't you ever mention the words "cancer" or "death" or "dying" in this house, or you won't be coming again.' It can make your work much more difficult.* Maggie Bisset, nurse consultant in palliative care

*As soon as my mother heard the word 'cancer', she fully expected to keel over the very next week, but she lived another 17 years and ended up dying from a completely different condition.* Rabbi Julia Neuberger

When I wrote an article recently for a major daily newspaper about lung cancer and how little public attention and research money it gets because people are thought to have brought the disease upon themselves, I was discussing the headline we might use with one of the sub-editors and suggested 'The cancer with the serves-you-right stigma'. 'Oh no,' said the sub, with an audible shudder. 'We couldn't possibly do that. You see, the editor won't have the word "cancer" in a headline.'

It's not just the non-medics among us who cannot bear to call it by its name. Even doctors and experts shy away from the word and tiptoe around, talking about 'the disease'.

*My oncologist refers vaguely to further courses of treatment that might be undertaken if I 'get into trouble again'.* Anna Blackman

Cancer is so hard to talk about, its presence in any sentence such an obscenity, that the person who breaks the news, nearly always the person with the illness, has the terrible task of saying 'the C-word'.

*In the days after the diagnosis, a friend would phone up and ask, as is the way of things, how I was. Sometimes I would forget how I was. I'd say, as one does, 'Fine, and you?' And then have to back-track because of course I wasn't fine. So I'd say, 'Actually, I say that, I say I'm fine, but, well, I've got cancer.'*

*What else can you say? You can't build up to it slowly – 'I'm, ill. No, not a cold: really ill. No: worse than flu. No, no: better than Aids but worse than flu. OK: two syllables.'* John Diamond, *C: because cowards get cancer too*

Often, our own shock and despair are redoubled by the emotions of those around us. We end up sparing the feelings of those closest to us, putting them at their ease, reassuring them, comforting them, cheering them up.

*When my best friend John Merritt was diagnosed with leukaemia, the first time he told me, he told me straight out, and then laughed and said, 'What a bummer eh?' Something like that. He had*

71

*already worked out that, having dealt with the big blow himself, it was up to him to try to soften the blow for family and friends. So he made light of it. Of course, nothing does soften the blow. But I went into 'It'll be OK' mode, prattling on about science and doctors and how great the NHS is, and he could see I was really upset and not wanting to show it, and I could see he was panicking but didn't want to show it.* Alastair Campbell

*At the moment, I'm regularly in and out of the Royal Marsden holding coffee mornings for the ladies with breast cancer for the thesis I'm writing for my psychology degree, and what comes across loud and clear from talking to them is that what very often causes most anxiety is not the cancer but the reactions of the people around them. As friends and family, we have to remember that this is a time when their needs absolutely must come first. We cannot inflict our own fears and anxieties on them. We have to give them space. It's not our emotional trip.* Ruby Wax

*I was so worried initially about telling my mum and my sisters, I thought, 'Gosh, how can I put them through this?' So I wasn't very forthcoming, I'd use this medical language that I didn't even understand myself. I'd say things like, 'I've just got to have this marginal clearance.' And I pulled away from them. Rather than being open and honest, there was this distance; it was my way of protecting myself from their fear and distress.* Nazira Visram

## WORDS AND QUESTIONS TO AVOID

• 'Riddled'/'terminal' (Implies the end is near. Try 'advanced', 'chronic' or 'recurrent', and then only if absolutely necessary.)

• 'God rest her soul' (After story of best friend's second-cousin thrice removed with supposedly similar cancer.)

• Clichés ('Cancer is a word not a sentence'; 'Any one of us could get run over by a bus tomorrow'; 'Life is a terminal disease'.)

• 'Look on it as a gift' (What did *you* get for Christmas?)

• 'If anyone can beat it, you can' (Nice to have a vote of confidence, but what a burden to place on even the healthiest of us.)

• 'What's your prognosis?'/'Is it terminal?'/'How long have you been given?'/'How did the scan go?' (All *very* intrusive. People living with cancer are often deeply superstitious about relaying the results of tests and scans, even when the news is good.)

• 'It's not surprising. You've always had such stressful jobs/relationships/life experiences' (Delete as appropriate.)

• 'It's not surprising. You've always had a bad relationship with your mother/your partner/yourself' (Delete as appropriate.)

73

- 'It's not surprising. You've always had difficulty expressing your emotions/anger/sorrow/fear' (Delete as appropriate.)

- 'I know how you're feeling' (You don't.)

- 'I know everything's going to be fine' (You don't.)

It may seem like a minefield – like 'walking on eggshells', as one person succinctly put it – but whatever you do, don't let the fear of saying the wrong thing deter you from saying anything at all. Confronted with the horror of a cancer diagnosis, some people take fright, back right off and avoid all contact. There was much more bitterness, sadness and anger among the people I talked to about the friends who had let them down by not being there at all, who had 'run for the hills' or crossed the road, than about those who had made insensitive or thoughtless comments.

*My response is to be in touch, to take them out to lunch, to reach out and not to cross the road because I don't know what to say, or to sit at home and say, 'How dreadful, poor thing.'* Felicia Williams

*My foul-weather friends were just fantastic. But there were a lot of peripheral people who were completely useless. They didn't write, they didn't ring, they didn't visit, they just did nothing because they didn't know what to do or, more to the point, what to say.* Charlie Wilson

# HOW TO BEHAVE WITH THE ILL

*Approach us assertively, try not to*
*cringe or sidle, it makes us fearful.*
*Rather walk straight up and smile.*
*Do not touch us unless invited,*
*particularly don't squeeze upper arms,*
*or try to hold our hands. Keep your head erect.*
*Don't bend down, or lower your voice.*
*Speak evenly. Don't say*
*'How are you?' in an underlined voice.*
*Don't say, 'I heard that you were very ill.'*
*This makes the poorly paranoid.*
*Be direct, say 'How's your cancer?'*
*Try not to say how well we look.*
*compared to when we met in Safeway's.*
*Please don't cry, or get emotional,*
*and say how dreadful it all is.*
*Also (and this is hard I know)*
*try not to ignore the ill, or to scurry*
*past, muttering about a bus, the bank.*
*Remember that this day might be your last*
*and that it is a miracle that any of us*
*stands up, breathes, behaves at all.*

Julia Darling

Be aware, be very aware, but try not to agonise later about what you might have said to give offence. In all the shock and anger following the diagnosis, it is common to be a bit prickly and hypersensitive. Those who did initially take offence at thoughtless comments later acknowledged that actually it was very hard and no one could get it right.

*I felt I needed extra sensitivity, and found it so hard dealing with my friends' fears and emotions on top of my own. At first I judged them quite harshly on how they responded – I was furiously put out, for example, when one of my more tactless friends lifted my hat up and asked, 'What's the hair situation like?' But recently I came round full circle when I had to deal with my dying friend's husband. I made some really stupid comments because I wanted to say SOMETHING, but was unsure what to say.* Georgie Hall

Doctors don't get it right, either. While some of the people I talked to reported being lost and confused by the medicalese, hating to ask for translations every few minutes ('Why don't they just talk plain English like the rest of us?'), others resented being talked down to. 'First on the helpful list must be doctors who recognise you might be able to understand an explanation even if you don't have a PhD in oncology.'

While there are inevitable differences in how certain approaches are received, here is a short list of things that were generally felt to be either helpful or the opposite:

**Helpful**

• 'Trivia, gossip, jokes.'

• 'Not minding when I don't make contact.'
'

• 'Understanding when I can't talk.'

• 'Having time when illness is not the subject.'

• 'Listening and not judging when I go on ceaselessly about symptoms, even when they've heard it all before.'

• 'Restoring a sense of normality.'

**Unhelpful**

• 'Making assumptions about how I'm feeling.'

• 'Telling me what will make me feel better and not listening to my opinions about what makes me feel better.'

• 'Asking "How *are* you?" in that oh-so-sepulchral, chapel-of-rest voice.'

• 'Demanding the nitty-gritty of the diagnosis or treatment by the school gates or over the phone, when children may be in earshot.'

• Bossiness, 'especially telling me what I should be doing to make myself better and why I got the cancer in the first place.'

• Tears, grief, panic, 'having to cope with other people's emotions on top of my own'.

• Me-too misery: 'having to smile through the minutiae of other people's unhappy marriages or hip-replacement operations'.

## 16. *Accept that you do not have to give advice. Listening is usually much more helpful*

Since we are all different, there can never be a single formula for the 'correct' response. Even so, it's usually not what you say that matters most, but how you listen. So relax, and rather than concentrating on what you should or shouldn't be saying, and attempting to provide answers, try listening instead. Equally, don't rush to fill the silences or stop the tears or bombard us with 'helpful' advice. We all know this is beyond your capacity to fix. Just be with us – without being afraid of our pain or our fear or our anger. If you don't change the subject or try to talk us out of these feelings, however huge and uncomfortable, your quiet acceptance is likely to mean more than any cheering words.

If today's visit is not the big heart-to-heart you were antici-pating, and it is clear that your arrival is a welcome distraction, then it is up to you to jump in with gossip and jokes and chat about anything and everything but the illness. On other days, however, your friend may need to talk. In fact, many people with cancer feel a compelling need to 'tell the tale' – not just once, but many times over.

Psychotherapists say that this is usually a necessary and healthy repetition: by telling and retelling our story, over and over and over again, we start to make sense of the shock and the trauma, to give it a place in the mind that's manageable, so that it can be thought about without sending us into a downward spiral of despair. We can then begin to feel more in control, even if the future is very uncertain.

At such times, give clues that you are not hurrying off and have as much time as is needed: sit down, take your coat off, offer to make tea, switch off your mobile phone. If you are unsure whether discussion of the illness is on the cards, say 'Do you feel like talking?' or 'I do want you to know that, if and when you do want to talk, I'm here to listen. It doesn't have to be today or next week or any time soon, but when you want to open up, I'll be here for you.'

*Tune in to what is being communicated, even if you feel you've heard it all before. Is there a new anxiety coming through? A new hopeful-ness? A sense of being traumatised all over again by the diagnosis or by the treatment? The story may seem the same, but the underlying feelings are often different. So don't assume you know what's coming. Recognise that every time the story is told, it becomes a way of trying to assimilate the overwhelming and bring it down to manageable proportions.* Natasha Harvey, psychoanalytic psychotherapist

*An interesting study took place in the United States in which a number of people were taught the simple techniques of good listening. Volunteer patients then came to see them to talk about their problems. The listeners in this study were not allowed to say or do anything at all. They just nodded and said 'I see' or 'Tell me more'. They weren't allowed to ask questions, or to say anything at all about the problems that the patients described. At the end of the hour, almost all of the patients thought they had got very good help and support – and some of them rang the 'therapists' to ask if they could see them again, and to thank them for the therapy.* From the CancerBACUP leaflet *Lost for Words*

Here are some simple but effective ways of signalling that you are ready to hear what your friend might want to say…

• Make sure you are somewhere private – not, for example, in a busy corridor or on the street.

• Check you are reasonably close, but not so close your friend feels hemmed in, and on a similar level and that there are no obstacles between you. Move furniture aside if necessary.

• Steel yourself for some strong emotions: we don't suddenly switch into serene, evolved beings – 'some kind of apprentice angel with a foot in two worlds', as one woman put it – in the wake of a cancer diagnosis. We may be full of anger, resentment, bitterness and fear. Be prepared to hear and acknowledge these feelings, however frightening or hard you find it, giving your full attention, without trying to deflect or contradict what your friend is saying, or rehearsing what you are going to say next.

• Make space for silences without filling them with words.

• Give encouragement by nodding and saying things like 'Yes', 'I see, and…?', 'And what happened next?' or 'Go on', prompting them to go into even more detail so they can explore the experience in more depth.

• Don't change the subject, even when you find what you are hearing very tough, very angry and very bitter.

• If what you are hearing is full of dread – 'The cancer has spread', 'I might die soon' – listen and try not to contradict. The best oncologists tune in to how patients are feeling every bit as attentively as they take note of a radiological report or an X-ray.

81

• Show you are listening in a spirit of acceptance by picking up on things your friend has said. This is called '*reflective listening*'.

> **HOW TO LISTEN REFLECTIVELY** Tune in to what your friend is saying, repeating words they have just said or picking words of your own that echo theirs – 'You must have felt devastated', 'Yes, I can see, just so fearful about what lay ahead' – indicating that you have heard their anxiety, apprehension or dread. The same skills can be used with our relatives and close friends.

*My friend Terry just sat and listened. I told him about my visit to the hospital and the doctor telling us that Naseem, my partner, had cancer. He looked right at me and told me he was shocked and he knew I was, too. He said, 'I expect you feel like your world is upside-down and you don't know what to do.' He was right and it was such a relief that he knew.* From the Macmillan Cancer Relief leaflet *Close Relationships and Cancer*

# 17. *Let your friend give you the lead about how much they want or don't want to talk about their illness*

Some people are intensely private, pull the bedclothes over their heads and prefer to face their demons alone; others broadcast their cancer to the world – sharing every last detail of their symptoms, treatment and results with an audience they don't know and have never even met via the internet. Most of us fall somewhere between these two extremes.

A friend of mine, Marianna Falconer, told me that for five years her sister-in-law Alice didn't tell a living soul that she had breast cancer, other than her own husband. 'In fact, she went to quite extraordinary lengths to hide it – telling one or other sibling that she was away when in fact she was in hospital having some operation or treatment. She later said that if she had told us, we would have treated her differently, and that what she wanted most of all was normality. She did not want anyone else's tears. She explained that she felt she was on a different planet after her diagnosis. And when the time came and she did tell us, however much we didn't want to treat her differently, we did.'

As Marianna found, you cannot assume the same degree of openness is appropriate on every occasion. 'Sometimes Alice wanted to talk and other times she did not. And what she helped me to understand is that sometimes I could help and other times I really could not. It did not mean she had gone off me or anything like that. Just that sometimes, much as she loved us, she was on that planet.'

*What I value from friends is acceptance of how I'm feeling at this moment. Sometimes I don't want to talk about it and other times I couldn't possibly talk about anything else. And a good friend is the person who'll say, 'Do you want to talk about it, mate?', and who'll accept that if you don't want to talk about it now, that's fine, but you might another time.* Ian Young, aged 45, diagnosed with a brain tumour five years ago (quoted by Joanna Moorehead, 'I don't know what to say', *The Guardian*, G2, 8 February 2005)

*At first I had a problem with knowing when they wanted to talk about it – the operation, the chemotherapy, the endless, endless blood tests – and when they didn't. I tried desperately to find a balance between seeming not to care enough and appearing a little too interested, morbid even. But slowly you get to spot when your daily 'Hello, how are you?' needs to be extended to 'Hello, how ARE you?' You just get a feeling that today is the day they want to say more than just 'I'm fine, thanks'. There are no rules, you just sort of get to know. You have to.* Nigel Slater

Even when cancer and possible death are no-go areas, the so-called 'elephant in the room' that no one can acknowledge but that is equally impossible to ignore, a little imagination and humour can often light the way through.

*My mother, who developed breast cancer in her seventies, didn't want the word mentioned, but she was a pushover when it came to jokes and, once she'd got the one about the favourite procedure of male medical students, was prepared to discuss her operation as another example of a Tube (Totally Unnecessary Breast*

*Examination) by a supposedly sex-obsessed surgeon. I know she was happy to find a way of talking about something that frightened her, but in truth I think it was laughing that was best for both of us. We still couldn't say 'cancer', though.* Andro Linklater

> **NB** Maggie Bisset, my palliative care nurse, has known some people who have used a pre-arranged code on days when they could not bear to talk about anything to do with their cancer. 'It could be "Let's leave that out in the garden" or "No sugar in my tea today" – something that's quick and non-threatening, and that can be used as a metaphor or symbol to flag a conversational no-go area.'

# 18. *Accept that comparative tales of other people with cancer are rarely helpful*

With hundreds of different types of cancer, and many different stages, it is rarely helpful to talk about other cases, since they almost certainly concern people of completely different ages with a completely different cancer in completely different circumstances. Two people who seem to have the same kind of cancer affecting the same part of the body may have quite distinct types of the disease and require alternative approaches to treatment.

85

Awful experiences of cancer are usually not just irrelevant; they are seriously depressing. Tales that don't have happy endings, or are prefaced with some gloomy fact about someone with advanced cancer 'who's been given six months to live', do not help us count our blessings. They are much more likely to add to the burden of gloom.

*For some reason, everyone talks about the people who didn't survive. I had two primary cancers, which was pretty unusual. And when I got the second one, people told me such terrible bad-news stories, they instigated fears that weren't there in the first place. I do remember with such gratitude one doctor saying to me, 'Two primaries? That's nothing. I've seen a patient with six.'* Sam Taylor-Wood

*I was struck by the wide range of responses, including being staggered by some well-meant stories of extreme pessimism. One person said, 'Oh, you've got breast cancer, my aunt died of it last year. She died so bravely.' I did not want to know about anyone who had died, however courageously. I wanted to hear about people who had survived.* Mary Allen

*Lots and lots of people were inspired to tell me stories about friends, relations who had had cancer, the trouble they had had getting diagnosed, the horror of the treatment, how they never went back to work again, and so on. I never knew how to react to these*

*stories. My sympathy reserves were low, and the diagnoses and*
*situations in these stories often bore no relevance to mine. More*
*alarmingly, the stories often petered out as it suddenly dawned on*
*the tellers that the punchline was that the person was now dead.*
Kate Carr, *It's Not Like That, Actually*

# 19. *Avoid false reassurances, which could be seen to make light of the cancer*

No one, sick or well, wants to dwell on the worst possibilities. Conversations and preoccupations that seem morbid and depressing are distressing. But the fact is that the fear accompanying cancer is real, and realistic, not an example of negative thinking that we can be jollied out of.

The prognoses may vary, but cancer is always a serious disease that brings with it disturbing intimations of mortality. Fears and forebodings should be acknowledged rather than denied with a glib reassurance or speedy change of subject. Please do your best to understand that we may feel the need to prepare for the worst, while also doing our utmost to secure the best possible outcome.

When I was concerned about the possible spread of my cancer, I found few friends prepared even to entertain the thought, let alone acknowledge the reality of my fear, as though merely to articulate this negative development would be enough to bring it about. Talking about the possibility or probability, even (my consultant would have said) certainty, of impending death was equally difficult. This meant that I was unable to share the things preying most upon my mind, apart from with a few dear, unfrightened individuals.

Friends would jump in with other explanations, which were intended to be reassuring but actually just intensified my feelings of isolation. No, no, they said, the increased breathlessness that I feared was due to steadily diminishing lung function was bound to be due to low haemoglobin caused by the chemotherapy, or because I wasn't as fit as I had been. Hell, they said, they couldn't go up the stairs without panting, either. The return of my headaches was due to the hypoxia (lack of oxygen) caused by, yes, you've guessed it, the low haemoglobin caused by...

As I didn't have the energy or strength or inclination to argue, I soon learnt to bring up these pressing, but depressing, subjects only with the few people who could bear to hear them. One work colleague, who I didn't know nearly as well as some of my other friends, was a tremendous source of solace, because she wasn't afraid. She would simply sit and hear what I was saying, adding observations of her own from time to time.

*Other [people] could not bear to talk about cancer at all and would stop all discussion with: 'I just know you're going to be fine.'*

*As my oncologist never said that to me, it was pretty galling to hear it from people who often would have been at a loss to explain exactly what an oncologist was.* Kate Carr, *It's Not Like That, Actually*

*The line 'You'll get better – I know you will' was bad enough when it was just a matter of recovering from a cyst, but when they were giving their judgement on throat cancer I started to get angry.*

*'John – it will be fine. I know it will.'*

*'How do you know?'*

*'Because I know you. You won't let it defeat you.'*

*'You know me? What, you know that I'm immortal? That I'm not susceptible to cancer like other people?'*

*'No, just that, well…'*

*It was unfair of me, I know. People say things because they don't know what to say, and they turn their wishes – that they don't want me to be ill, to be frightened, to die – into statements of fact.* John Diamond, *C: because cowards get cancer too*

# 20. *Try to fit your response to the person, not to the preconceptions you may have*

The contemporary emphasis on positive thinking can place a real burden on everyone – not just the person with cancer, but families, friends and visitors alike – to be forever upbeat. This look-on-the-bright-side optimism may be just what the doctor ordered for some of us, but others are likely to find the pressure of putting on a constant *faux*-cheeriness at cruel odds with the heart-twisting horror of their situation. Try to put yourself in their place, and you will soon see that remaining resolutely cheerful and 'positive' is a tall order when you've just been told you have a life-threatening disease and are, quite possibly, facing some very unpleasant treatment ahead.

*People try to cheer you up. 'It's not that bad,' they say. 'At least it's treatable.' But when it's the worst thing that's ever, ever happened to you, it's hard to look on the bright side.* Alan Straker

*The bloke that went cycling, the bloke that won the Grand National: we've got a whole shelf of inspirational titles, and a thoroughly depressing one it is, too.* Sarah Poland

*One decision I made early on was to ignore all the 'positive attitude' merchants who suddenly started targeting me by letter and telephone. 'You must think positive,' they told me, as if it was some great secret only they were privy to – as if, without their important insight, I would be smearing myself with ashes and rolling in the dunghill. For most of them, I suspected, it was just a convenient way to wash their hands of you and your problems. Have a 'positive attitude' and you can defeat anything. Drop dead, and it's obviously your own fault for not being positive enough.* Martyn Harris, 'This is not the time to die', *The Spectator,* 19 August 1995

*There have been many articles and books written about long-term cancer survivors, about how, looking back, cancer has in some way redefined their lives, even to the point of giving them a feeling of gratitude for their illness. Lance Armstrong's It's Not About the Bike is one. Such positive attitudes are inspirational for us all, but sometimes I long to hear from others who are battling less brilliantly, who say how hard this path can be, and who acknowledge that being unremittingly cheerful is just not possible.* Sally Hamilton

*My three good friends and one favourite aunt who have developed breast cancer have taught me that the important thing is simply to be there for them. To try to be the person with whom they can express whatever they want or need without worrying about how it sounds; without feeling they have to be strong and brave or you will somehow think less of them. As a friend, I need to be able to hear all this, without communicating how terrible and awful I feel, and without assuming this is their definitive 'take' on the disease. It's just what they feel today.*

*There's no point in pretending. So many people with cancer feel they don't have the permission to be fearful or downcast or sad or even defeated. They worry that any 'negativity' will frighten their friends away or concern their family or jeopardise their survival chances. They shouldn't have to worry about these things, to put a brave face on. They should be able to do what they need to do and say what they need to say. And the rest of us should be able to cope with it.* Cherie Blair

## 21. *One gut-wrenching diagnosis is plenty, so leave it there*

It's human nature to seek a cause for the things that happen to us, and this is especially so when cancer strikes because of all the powerful and widespread myths that attach to it. Namely, that stress or the 'toxic' emotions that we have repressed, such as grief or anger, can somehow cause cells to mutate. As Woody Allen said, 'I don't get angry. I grow tumours instead.'

Many of the authors of the cancer memoirs I read or the people I spoke to when putting this book together said they were assaulted by well-meaning people who were determined to help them to see what they had done to give themselves cancer. 'Those who couldn't bear to contemplate the idea that it was simply bad luck that I had cancer tried to find a very specific reason why I had it and, therefore, why they wouldn't get it,' wrote Kate Carr in *It's Not Like That, Actually*. 'It was often implied that it was my fault.'

Whether this amateur psychologising springs from fear or misinformation, or the belief that those of us who suffer in some Job-like way deserve it or that we have 'bad karma' (to use a New Ageism), it takes a strong degree of self-confidence to reject suggestions that we find harmful or disempowering, that make us feel afraid and guilty, especially if we already feel that in some way we may indeed be to blame for our predicament.

It may be only natural to search for meaning, and if we who have the cancer are keen to explore such ideas, then please feel free to come along for the ride. But even then, be wary of coming up with half-baked theories of your own. If you are spinning theories, you are not saying 'I love you, I care about you, what can I do to help?' but 'Now let's see what you did to bring this cancer on yourself. What did you do wrong?'

When I myself was told by some self-appointed amateur psychologist that 'You do know, don't you, that the lungs are the centre of grief?', I was gobsmacked by her presumption. I let my interlocutor know in no uncertain terms that, actually, I attributed my illness to the deadly combination of a rubbish gene (two first-degree relatives died of lung cancer), an early smoking habit, and exposure to tobacco smoke in infancy.

A good friend of mine, the writer Guillermo Gil, points out: 'If the theory about the link between cancer and emotional repression had any merit, by now, when people tell each other everything, go to the gym, have sex without logistical or ethical problems, and therapists are as available as hairdressers and, if all else fails, they can call a radio phone-in or take part in reality-TV shows, cancer rates should have plummeted – which is not the case.'

93

*I was lying in a hospital bed, recovering from both the news that I had cancer and the radical operation to remove it, when I was stunned to receive a visitor whose opening remark was 'I wouldn't have thought YOU'D be the type to get cancer.' That was back in the 1980s, when theories about repressed emotions kick-starting tumours were very fashionable. I knew it was all nonsense, but I still felt apologetic, as though the cancer were in some way my fault and I was paying the price for having brought such a catastrophe upon myself.* John Anderson

*When other people apply their rules to you, it's very difficult to take. I learnt to say 'Fuck off'. It was hard enough for myself to try and fathom it without having to take everyone else's crackpot theories on board.* Sam Taylor-Wood

*You do get some crap thrown at you. My cancer probably originated in the pancreas, so I was told that this was due to a poor relationship with my mother. Rubbish. I had a good relationship with my mother… Now I just take the bits that suit me. For example, I like the theories that being happy is good for the immune system, so I feel good about indulging myself with lots of treats, like going to the cinema in the afternoon.* Suzanne Long

*I have had cancer. I feel bad enough about this, about the threat to my life, about the surgery and treatments I have had to undergo. It has been frightening. I have felt guilty for getting cancer. I have*

94

*asked myself what I might have done to bring this on myself. I have been unkind to myself in asking some of these questions. Please help. I do not need you to be unkind to me too. I need you to understand, to be gentle, to help me wrestle with these questions. I do not need you to theorise about me behind my back, so to speak. I need you to ask me, not to tell me. I need you to try to understand what this must feel like, just a little, to put yourself in my place and hopefully treat me more kindly than I sometimes treat myself.*
Treya Killam Wilber, *Grace and Grit*

## 22. *Accept that denial can be both positive and necessary*

The notion that there is a set number of psychological stages following a diagnosis of cancer also has a strong hold on the contemporary psyche – the notion being that we embark on a cancer 'journey', moving from a state of out-and-out denial, through anger, bargaining and grief, to a Zen-like, calm acceptance. Some unwise types who subscribe a little too faithfully to these ideas may bring it upon themselves to try to bring a friend out of denial by forcing conversations they are not ready for. Even if you feel your friend is failing to acknowledge the seriousness of the diagnosis and its potential outcome, denial can be a very useful coping mechanism and, in the bleakness following diagnosis, may appear to be the only way forward. Respect it.

*I do not believe I'm in denial, but maybe that's what denial is. If not letting it rule my life is denial – I don't know, I'm not sure that denial is actually bad. I think you can accept certain realities, but you don't need to force them on yourself. I don't wake up every morning and say, 'Oh my God, I'm dying of lung cancer.' I view myself as living with lung cancer, which is a different thing altogether. I emotionally acknowledge that statistically it is very likely to kill me, and there are days when I think this is a bit of a bugger, frankly, but you can't stop it. I can't sit at home being miserable, so I don't.* Nick Baker, aged 46, insurance-broker and cross-Atlantic yachtsman and fundraiser (quoted by Penny Wark, 'A buoyant approach', *The Times*, T2, 31 January 2005)

# During
# treatment

This is a time when the need for help may either temporarily
fall off or intensify; so be sensitive as to whether this is the
moment to back off and put your energies into supporting
the principal care team, or to roll up your shirtsleeves and get
really stuck in.

## 23. *Support any decision 110 per cent*

After all the anxiety of having to weigh the various options for treatment, it can be a big relief to make the decision to go ahead with a particular strategy. This chosen course needs to be wholeheartedly supported by family and friends. What is emphatically not needed at this point are questions or reservations or information about alternative routes that cast doubt on the wisdom of proceeding with the proposed option.

*In the end you make your decision, trust in your consultant and go for it. You can drive yourself mad otherwise. Wondering should you, shouldn't you, what are the alternatives, as we did at the beginning, caused a lot of anxiety. The thought that you may not be being offered the right treatment is a huge worry; and, with the best will in the world, friends can really play on that. To find someone you trust, and you can hand over your care to, is such a relief. It helps take away from that feeling of being the victim.* Heidi Locher

## 24. *Draw up a list together of useful things to take to hospital*

If friends are going to be staying a few nights, it's helpful to take things that will help to enhance their sense of well-being.

Not just the obvious (pyjamas, dressing gown, slippers, sponge-bag, hairbrush, toothbrush and toothpaste, shampoo), but also those small non-essentials that make any time away from home just that little bit more comfortable:

- Spare pairs of pyjamas/nighties.

- Special soap, scent and air-freshener.

- Books and magazines.

- A box of tissues.

- Alarm clock with illuminated numbers for checking the time in the still watches of the night.

- Loose change for phone/newspapers, etc.

- Wax earplugs to drown out the sound of other people snoring.

- A home duvet and pillow to replace the NHS standard issue.

- Address book, pen and paper.

- A bottle of a cordial, such as elderflower or pink ginger, does wonders for the taste of hospital water.

## 25. *Be sensitive when visiting. Do not overstay your welcome*

Make it known when you can visit (including if you can be called to come in at short notice) so that the partner/primary support person can put together a visitor rota.

*I was known as 'the ogre', having had to clamp down on visits fairly early on after 17 people turned up for a drinks party on Liddy's balcony at the Wellington!* Peter Gwilliam

Being sociable is exhausting for people who are not well, but they will often not have the strength to ask you to go, or will not want to offend you by doing so. Be an undemanding presence. Bring something to occupy you (tapestry, knitting, sewing, a newspaper) that takes away the obligation of having to talk or, worse, entertain. Offer to leave after half an hour, and if your friend does not beg you to stay, beat a swift retreat.

*Don't stay too long: 20 minutes is a good visit. Offer to change or wash nighties and pyjamas. Change the water for the flowers. Bring tiny nosegays – even daisies. Kiss hands, not always faces, and don't wear too much scent. Tell them you love them and smile as you go (if you can; if you can't, pretend that you're sneezing).* Joanna Lumley

If your friend is emphatic about not wanting visits at all, respect that too.

*I had this 10-hour operation to remove and reconstruct my bladder, and when I came to I counted 14 drips coming in and drains coming out, and I was in intensive care for a week. We agreed it would not be helpful for the children to come and see me. And I didn't want visitors. I was happier on my own.*
Charlie Wilson

# 26. *If visitors are not wanted, keep the letters and cards and emails going*

If you can't be there in person, get writing. Small notes with funny stories, wacky cards, witty observations, news clippings and newsy letters are all very sustaining; when feeling sick and weak, it's especially nice to know one is being thought about, that people still love and care even if they cannot be in direct contact.

*Liddy loved to know that people were enquiring, caring etc, even if not speaking to her directly. The most effective contact was via email. When she was having in-patient treatment, I would send out a group update saying that I was departing shortly to see her at whichever hospital and request emails within the hour. These would then pile in for me to take in and read out to her, to her tremendous pleasure.* Peter Gwilliam

## 27. *Offer to help transporting family*

Spending long hours in hospitals with loved ones is very draining, especially when they are gravely ill and relying on just one or two people to be with them, more or less full-time. Friends can do a huge amount to help: not only with transport to and from the hospital (likely to be especially appreciated if relying on public transport), but also by accompanying them into the house and helping to draw the curtains, switch on the lights, before sharing a cup of tea or a glass of wine to ease the loneliness.

*I was always very wary of driving down the A3 late at night – having tucked Liddy up in bed at the Royal Free Hospital at nearly midnight after a day at the bedside, knowing that I would have to be back in the morning after the school run. The simple offer from drivers living nearby to drive me back, stay the night and drive me into London again, was hugely helpful.* Peter Gwilliam

*During my husband's stay in hospital following a fairly serious cancer op, I was driving 20 miles to and from the hospital –*

*often twice a day. I was finding myself tired and stressed by these journeys, so it was wonderful when a friend offered to do some of the runs. It was not only relaxing to be driven, but so nice to have company and to chat about topics other than my husband's illness, which I was rather inclined to dwell on when alone.*
Joyce Cormie

## 28. *Find out helpful information about the proposed chemotherapy regime and avoid recycling horror stories*

There are many different types of chemotherapy, all with different side effects (the CancerBACUP database lists 50 individual drugs and 28 different combination regimes alone), and people vary hugely in their responses to them. Since everybody's experiences and levels of tolerance are different, and chemotherapy probably has the worst press of any medical treatment, forewarned is rarely forearmed – just terrified.

I was personally amazed by one well-meaning friend who went into such lurid descriptions about what I could expect from my soon-to-be-embarked-upon course of chemotherapy, you would have thought she was describing a Quentin Tarantino horror movie or the shock-and-awe campaign of the Iraq war. The reality, I was amazed to find, was quite different.

Where was the sickness? The fatigue? The hair coming out in hanks on my pillow? The mouth ulcers and tremors and fevers? I was lucky, my type of chemotherapy turned out to be particularly tolerable, and I tolerated it very well. But so do many people, and their stories are seldom told.

*I knew nothing about chemotherapy, what it was or how it was administered. I just had the idea that it was the worst the medical profession could throw at you. What I quickly discovered was that it was the best the medical profession could throw at you despite the fact there were no guarantees that it would destroy all the possible cancer cells in my body.* Kate Carr, *It's Not Like That, Actually*

*I can only describe the worst of it as a combination of the mother of all hangovers, seasickness and flu all at once... But although those days are rough, the human spirit and memory are amazing. It only takes one good day (like today) to put a whole different perspective on things and you realise you can make it through; it is just a case of grinning and bearing it. Maybe I am a simple soul, but once I've had a pizza, a glass of wine, chocolate cake and a glass of Bushmills, I really feel quite good. There is light at the other end of the tunnel and, in hindsight, even the bad days don't seem so bad.* James Ewins

*I got used to the fact that there were good days and bad days. Good*

*days were defined by being out of bed with clean hair and a nice cup of tea. If I made it out for a coffee or herb tea with a friend, that was a bonus.* Sally Hamilton

> **NB** Help your friend to know what to expect from a given regime, bearing in mind that individuals respond very differently even to identical forms of treatment, by going to CancerBACUP's website www.cancerbacup.org.uk (click on 'Treatment', then on 'Chemotherapy' and 'Individual drugs' or 'Combination regimes').

# 29. *Offer to be an outpatient companion...*

At its best, this entails accompanying your friend from their front door and back again, helping them on and off public transport or, better, in and out of cars and taxis, and doing whatever you can to minimise hassle, such as distances to be walked, fares to be paid and things to be carried. Radiotherapy sessions rarely last more than a few minutes (though the waiting can be another matter), whereas chemotherapy sessions can often last several hours.

Bring a selection of things that will make the latter more pleasant (a Thermos flask of coffee or soup, some home-made biscuits) and amusing: crosswords, puzzles, a game, such as

Scrabble or chess, that you can play together, even a portable DVD player for super-long sessions. One old schoolfriend of mine brought in a batch of letters we had written each other as boy-mad 14-year-olds and the time seemed to go in the blink of an eye, with much mutual reminiscing and laughter.

A friend can also be a great support by offering to go out for a better class of coffee, soup or sandwich than can be had on the cash-strapped NHS, and by acting as a mediator between the patient and the nursing team, making requests that the patient might find hard to do. It is often much easier, for example, to negotiate more convenient chemotherapy or radiotherapy appointments that fit better with one's lifestyle and schedule if you are doing it on someone else's behalf.

Friends can also do much to alleviate some of the minor traumas of treatment. One woman I know remains eternally gratefully to the forthright friend who had noticed that, as often happens as chemotherapy continues, her friend's veins had hardened and were becoming more and more difficult to find. Understandably, she came to dread the beginning of each session when the time came to put the needle in, flinching visibly if it was one of the nurses who somehow managed to make it hurt each time and who needed two or even three attempts to find the vein. From experience, this woman knew that there is always one nurse who has that magic talent for finding the vein first time. So she went and asked the sister in charge to make a specific note that this nurse should put in the line each time her friend came in, thus alleviating a huge amount of anxiety before every subsequent session.

*My brother, who had pancreatic cancer, was very clear about one thing. He always wanted someone with him when he was going to the hospital for his chemotherapy sessions. It sounds easy enough, but we actually found many of his friends making excuses or even cancelling at the last minute. This mystified us until we realised that they were actually frightened rather than merely unreliable, imagining chemotherapy to be a gruelling affair, with people hooked up to very toxic, very dangerous drugs, and a general air of terror.*

*The first time I accompanied my brother, the thing that struck me most forcibly was how calm and friendly and civilised it all was. People had popped in with their shopping, or were chatting to each other or eating sandwiches while hooked up to drips, and stands. None of them looked particularly ill. I thought they could have easily been under the dryers at my local hair salon.*
Anne-Sophie Capel

*There were times when I just wanted to be completely on my own so I could feel sorry for myself. At others, having company definitely distracted from the self-pity, especially when I was hooked up to a drip having chemotherapy. Some really good friends ran a rota and would take it in turns to put together a picnic every time I had chemo. They'd bring food and drink, really take trouble. Sometimes*

107

*it would just be one. Sometimes two or three. On the last session about six of them came for a bit of a party. But unfortunately it was a really traumatic session and I had to send them all away.*
Sam Taylor-Wood

## *… but don't press the point; some people prefer to undergo treatment alone*

*Two London friends came to sit with me for my first chemo session, but after that I discouraged other offers, preferring to see people when I felt better, and to have them keep in touch by email, letter, telephone and the like.*

*Time becomes so precious when you are having treatment that I would really rather just get the chemo done, and rest or deal quietly with the essentials and give any extra to my family, since there is so little energy for anything else. Now the chemo is over, I am spending time building new relationships, and all I really want from old friends and new is to be able to lead my life as normally as possible.*

*So when I don't feel well, I keep my head down and nobody need know – I prefer it that way. I see the bad bouts like childbirth – awful at the time, but soon forgotten once they have passed.*
Suzanne Long

## CHEMOTHERAPY

*I did not imagine being bald*
*at forty four. I didn't have a plan.*
*Perhaps a scar or two from growing old,*
*hot flushes. I'd sit fluttering a fan.*

*But I am bald, and hardly ever walk*
*by day. I'm the invalid of these rooms,*
*stirring soups, awake in the half dark,*
*not answering the phone when it rings.*

*I never thought that life could get this small,*
*that I would care so much about a cup,*
*the taste of tea, the texture of a shawl,*
*and whether or not I should get up.*

*I'm not unhappy. I have learnt to drift*
*and sip. The smallest things are gifts.*

Julia Darling

# 30. *Give a useful present*

• Flowers and plants – even better if they arrive in vases or planted baskets (to avoid having to find homes for them) as so much more time is spent at home than usual.

• A microfibre hair towel, 'so that I could help to protect against too much hair loss by avoiding excessive drying'.

• A footbath borrowed from a local pedicurist, some of those lovely aromatherapy foot products, and your services as a foot masseur.

• Chewing-gum to get rid of that horrid mouth taste.

• Silk pyjamas, generously cut, front-buttoning for post-mastectomy patients, when arm movement may be restricted. 'Again and again I bless them, the way they slide on, so cool, so soft, the dull, expensive sheen on them,' says Dina Rabinovitch.

• A soft, loose top or pair of trousers for wearing at home when undergoing radiotherapy, as the skin on the treated area may get very sore and fitted clothes quickly become uncomfortable.

• Cashmere bed socks.

• A plate of freshly cut chilled raw vegetables to cut through the depressing monotony of hospital food (carrots, pepper, celery) and dips (taramasalata, hummus, tzatziki, salsa).

• Home-made freshly squeezed and chilled ginger fruit juice, and ginger ale for relieving the effects of nausea – 'the only thing I found that got rid of the metallic taste in my mouth'.

• A couple of acupuncture sessions – for relieving the nausea.

• A 'chillow' – a cooling pillow filled with tap water (room temperature is below body temperature), perfect for easing the sunburn-like side effects of radiotherapy and for breast/ovarian/prostate cancer patients suffering hot flushes from hormone-based therapies (telephone 08700 117174 for mail order).

• A home massage – some hospitals now have in-house masseurs, so ask. 'When you have cancer and people are examining you in a very clinical way,' says palliative care nurse Maggie Bisset, 'it can be tremendously therapeutic to be touched in a way that has nothing to do with disease. That goes for friends, too. We all differ in what we feel comfortable with, but people often miss being touched affectionately.'

• A fabulous scarf to create a turban, or beanie hat for keeping bald heads warm. Specialist suppliers and details of how to tie scarves and turbans can be found in CancerBACUP's leaflet *Coping With Hair Loss.*

• A couple of aloe vera plants for use on unbroken radiation-sore skin. 'Once I was allowed to apply something direct to my skin, a good friend arrived with an aloe vera plant. It needed very little attention, and breaking open the stalks and holding them on to the skin like a poultice gave miraculous relief.'

• A talking book, for when you're too tired to open your eyes.

*Since I am an actress, and one of my jobs is recording books on tape, I like sending some of the tapes to my sick chums. Often people undergoing chemo or radiation treatment are very tired; they don't want to talk for hours on the phone, haven't the strength to hold a book or magazine, or the mental energy to concentrate. But if a nurse or family member can set up a CD player and put on the headphones, then my dulcet tones reading a good yarn can cheer them up, take their mind off cancer. A laugh is therapeutic. There are some wonderful BBC tapes: Round the Horne or Blackadder or The Wordsmiths of Gorsemere. Lots to choose from and it doesn't HAVE to be me reading them. Martin Jarvis reading the Just William stories is one of the world's wonders. And if they get tired, they can switch off and turn it on tomorrow.* Miriam Margolyes

## 31. *Try not to take fright at the physical changes. Keep up the compliments and use your ingenuity*

For many, women especially, the loss of one's hair, or the first sight of one's battle-scarred post-operative body, is the brutal moment of truth, when the reality of cancer hits with its most unforgiving force. Although my own cancer was unfortunately too advanced for surgery, and I weathered the chemotherapy without losing my hair, I still shrank from the gruesome vision of my reflection in the mirror. Having lost two stone in the space of just four months, I hated seeing the jutting clavicles and hipbones, visible ribs, bumpy vertebrae and wide-apart pelvic girdle with gaping space between the thighs that reminded me of nothing so much as a Holocaust victim.

I have always loved clothes, and ruefully surveying the items in my wardrobe that I had persuaded myself I would never again be able to wear because they were literally falling off me, a friend of mine with rather more common sense than I had came to the rescue with a box of pins and took about half a dozen skirts and trousers to the local dry-cleaners to have their waistbands taken in. Four days later, I was able to reclaim my wardrobe and, because everything now fitted, I felt 100 per cent better.

Like me, many women cannot bear to look at their diseased or surgically altered bodies, bald heads and lack of eyelashes. It took my mother months to summon up the courage to look at her colostomy, and even after 12 years she still finds it hard. People with cancer, both men and women (see Martyn Harris's quote below), are also super-quick to see revulsion or shock in the eyes of their friends. In *It's Not Like That, Actually*, the journalist Kate Carr, who didn't wear her wig at home because she found it unbearably claustrophobic and itchy, wrote that she would shout 'Bald!' at the top of her voice before opening the front door, giving advance warning that she hoped would protect her from the shocked looks she might otherwise have to endure.

In such situations, you can do nothing better than to treat your friends with total acceptance, giving women, especially, nurturing treats that make them feel feminine and desirable. One friend spoke gratefully of her partner, who 'made me feel beautiful even when my hair fell out'; another of the person who persuaded her to let her take photographs before and after the surgery she had feared would be so disfiguring, and enabled her to see how normal-looking her body still was; another of the friend she hardly knew who visited her at her bedside with a footbath and proceeded to carry out a pedicure. 'It was a marvellous treat to be able to look down and see sparkling little toenails winking cheery pink kisses at me – and no pain relief required.' Yet another lauded the friend, who had also been through chemotherapy, who advised her to have her hair cut short in stages, and to wear a hairnet at night to minimise the trauma of finding her hair on the pillow the following morning.

*I hated it, particularly when my hair fell out, and not just the hair on my head. I had no eyelashes, no eyebrows. A friend who had been through it came with the most enormous bundle of turbans and showed me how to tie them, but I didn't like them, I didn't want to look like Jane Russell. So I wore a wig, but, even so, there was nothing I could do to disguise the hairlessness on my face, that naked look that tells people you are having treatment for cancer and that marks you out.* Anna Blackman

*Two weeks after the first chemotherapy, all my hair fell out, which was the first real test of friends and relations. Up until then, the cancer had just been a horrible new fact, but now I was visibly the cancer victim, with the stigmata of raw pink scalp, absent eye-lashes. I made a point of telling people on the phone to prepare themselves before they came to see me, but most of them – men in particular – did not handle it well. They avoided looking at me, made jokes about Duncan Goodhew, said it would soon grow back. Women, on the other hand, seemed to make an effort to imagine themselves into my position before meeting me, and I seldom saw shock on their faces.* Martyn Harris, 'This is not the time to die', *The Spectator*, 19 August 1995

*The surgery, the hair loss, the pronounced weight loss or (as is some-times the case with breast-cancer treatments) gain can strike a real blow to a woman's self-image. I like to tell my friends how good they're looking, not in an empty, flattering way, but in a way that encourages them to believe they can still be attractive, that they are attractive, and to boost that in little practical ways – whether by passing on information about where to get the best wigs or giving small glamorous presents, such as fabulous scarves and make-up,*

115

*that acknowledge they are still one of the girls, and still care, often a great deal, about how they look.* Cherie Blair

*I was shell-shocked by the mastectomy. Chemotherapy hadn't knocked me out – the sickness and fatigue seemed familiar, like pregnancy nausea and post-baby exhaustion. But the bruising and immobility from the surgery were frightening. I felt invalided – not a condition I recognised. And I couldn't get dressed. Too sore to wear a bra, too angry to stuff some bit of foam down one, should I put one on.*

*Fiona Golfar from Vogue came to my rescue. We met just 10 days after I left hospital. She watched me struggle in and out of clothes, she racked her brains, and came up with Pleats Please, a Japanese idea: stretchy, pleated material, easy to put on even when your arms won't go over your head, and material that ripples over the body, creating shape even where new hollows lie.*

*Why did the clothes matter so much? They returned to me what the treatment for this illness took away – my looks.* Dina Rabinovitch

*Richard was very tender, loving my body and my scars. He made me feel very beautiful through it all, very sensual. It was very important to me to feel I was still attractive. Even at my sickest, it was important to me that I looked as good as I could. I wanted my hair washed and the lippy on. I'd be cross if the consultant came in too early, before I felt ready to be seen.* Heidi Locher

## 32. *Be sensitive that arrangements may have to be cancelled at short notice*

All the people I spoke to who had been through gruelling cancer treatments were united on one thing: don't fight the fatigue. If they resisted the urge to rest and went out, or entertained visitors when their energy levels were at rock bottom, they lived to regret it the next day. When undergoing treatment for cancer, all the best-laid plans can go quickly awry. So be ready to be cancelled at the last minute or, conversely, to be called upon at short notice to do something if your friend is feeling stronger than expected and up for some fun. And never visit without checking first.

*When my wife Anna was having her chemo and radiotherapy, we kept our social life much quieter than usual. But occasionally we'd accept an invitation to go out and if, on the day, she was feeling too exhausted to drag herself out, I soon learnt to ring and say, 'I'm sorry we can't come', and people were incredibly understanding, even if we rang only a couple of hours before we were due to arrive.*
Nigel Blackman

*In the Muslim community you support people in prayers. If someone is sick, it is your duty to visit them, to say a prayer for them. Yet I had been told I should keep away from people with germs. I*

117

*had to learn to be honest. I'd say, 'Can you please enquire before you come round?' Rather than just saying 'Don't come' and people getting offended, I'd explain that I'd been advised by a medical professional. That was more acceptable.* Nazira Visram

## 33. *Plan a project together around the experience*

It may be raising consciousness about your friend's particular cancer, or fundraising for a national charity or equipment for a local hospital (*Calendar Girls*-style), or encouraging them to write about the experience, either in blog form or a private diary or log (very cathartic), or even setting up a support group. In all the awfulness, it helps to feel that something constructive may one day come out of the experience.

*When I was discharged, the notion of any care in the community turned out to be mythical. There was no support whatsoever. So I founded a support group with my daughters. And it helped us every bit as much as the people who came along in their own turn.* Mary O'Brien

*When I sat for those endless hours in the chemo suite every week, I wrote a log of how people had responded, because not only was it very touching and excellent at improving my spirits, but also the*

*response from people frequently reflected their own personalities.*
Suzanne Long

*We did it to find a distraction, to find something besides the cancer, to make a project out of it. It gave me the idea that the project would have an ending and the ending would be that she was better, so it made me more hopeful. It also made it easier to look at her, to be by her side and see all the changes she was going through, to really be involved but to remain objective about it. It would have been really hard to stand by and not do anything.* Annabel Clark (quoted in the London *Evening Standard*, 8 March 2005), who photographed her mother, Lynn Redgrave, on her journey through breast cancer and out the other side for their book, *Journal: a mother and daughter's recovery from breast cancer*

*When they found the second primary in my colon, I was doing an MA in Fine Art at Central St Martins, painting empty spaces and still lives, and as I went through surgery and chemotherapy I decided that rather than sitting on the sofa feeling sorry for myself, I would paint my way through it, record what was happening and how I was feeling. Even though the tiredness and sickness and blurry vision compromised the amount of work I could do – and the quality, too, sometimes – my work went off in this totally new direction. I'd paint my face yellow and my eyes black to suggest the nausea of chemotherapy, or stitch sutures on to canvas, or make death's heads, or sculpt myself in boxes like coffins. At home I was*

119

*being so positive, so sunny, so absolutely not the victim, but in my studio I could explore all that anxiety and fear, all those morbid preoccupations.* Heidi Locher

## 34. *Plan treats ahead, so there's always something to look forward to*

Friends can help hugely here. What's required are two sorts of goals: small goals for the immediate future (whisking the children out of the house for a sleepover, facilitating a long soak in a candlelit bath and an early night; an aromatherapy massage session; fresh asparagus for supper) and bigger ones that may have to wait until the treatment is over, or things are looking a little more certain.

Make a plan of what you might plant together in the garden: trees (a real vote of confidence in the future) or rose bushes or vegetable plants. Even at the grimmest point, it can raise the spirits to look ahead to a time when your friend might be feeling well enough to visit that faraway place they've always fancied going, to watch some key sports fixture, or to visit children or grandchildren.

*A friend of mine had just finished having chemotherapy for breast cancer when I heard that Eric Clapton was playing at the Albert Hall. It was September and the concert was in March, so I bought*

*tickets for both of us, and the time rolled round and we went to the concert. And later, much later, she said, 'I can't thank you enough. I could never tell you at the time how important it was that you bought those tickets, because it meant you thought I'd still be alive in six months' time.' That was 11 years ago, and she's still in the best of health.* Anna Blackman

*A physician friend of mine with rectal cancer has a passion for music and travel. Every few weeks a friend of his would send him a CD with the music of a different part of the world, along with a video of a country he wanted to visit. He would have his chemo and listen to the CD, watch the video and plan his trips. He has been able to do some of them.* Robbie Alexander

*When my friend was diagnosed with cancer, one of the first things we did was to confirm the bookings for a shared summer holiday our families had talked loosely about. At times the holiday looked all but impossible, but everyone remained committed and it became an almost emblematic light at the end of the chemo tunnel.* Jon Snow

**NB** Presents that promise a return to a previous way of life or hobby or interest can be very cheering: fitness gear, a selection of bulbs for planting (plus planting services), fruit trees or flowering plants, a compass and sturdy pair of walking boots, a ski hat, a holiday brochure, haircare products or an eyebrow-shaping appointment for when the hair grows back.

121

# Practicalities

When someone gets cancer, people often imagine that what's required is a soul-baring heart-to-heart. But when one's world has just been turned upside-down, and there's a scary new schedule of appointments and consultations and treatments to be accommodated, it's often help with the logistics that's more useful – saying, for example, 'Give me your laundry basket and I'll do the ironing' or 'Can I do the family shop or take the kids to school/ballet/karate every Wednesday?' or 'Let me drive you to the hospital/find out about holiday insurance/set up a group email that will keep us all informed so you don't have to keep on repeating yourself'. Just one or two things to lighten the load will help to establish a return to normality; something those of us living with cancer yearn for more than anything else.

*When you are in hospital people say, 'Don't do this', 'Don't do that', and then you get home and there is a pile of ironing or the groceries to put away, or the saucepans to be put on the hob. I had had a mastectomy and lymph-node clearance in my right armpit, and was told to be very careful about using my right arm in order to prevent this condition where your whole side can swell up. So I had to be really careful and do everything with my left hand, right down to brushing my teeth and filling the kettle. As I'm a single mother, I was so grateful to my friend who came in and did the children's ironing and the neighbour who never complained whenever I rang him to lift things that needed lifting or to take the casserole out of the oven.* Sandra Lilley

*Intensive radiotherapy knocked the stuffing out of me. I was so, so exhausted, I'd burst into tears without a reason, couldn't cope with noise, couldn't rest without feeling guilty, cranky, unsociable. I needed to cook but couldn't bring myself to do it, so I would worry about what we were going to eat. It took me a long time to be open and honest, to admit I wasn't fine and to help myself recover by getting the support I desperately needed.* Nazira Visram

123

Be sensitive that your helpfulness is not seen as 'taking over'. Always ask first. If offers of help are not readily accepted, it may be that your friend really does prefer to do it for the time being. When we have cancer, and our life seems to be careering out of control, most of us need to feel that we can keep a grip on at least some of it; that we amount to more than useless invalids. Even though, at particularly difficult times, we might need to pass that control over to a close friend or relative, we are likely to want to reclaim our responsibilities as soon as we feel well enough to do so.

While there is nothing better than the sort of ongoing support that can be counted on week in, week out, the disappointment of being let down at the last minute, and having to take over ourselves or find replacements when we may be feeling unwell and disinclined to ask for further favours, can be crushing. It is essential, therefore, not to promise more than you feel you can deliver, and to recognise that help might be most welcome in those months when treatment is over and all those well-intentioned offers of support have trickled away – which is exactly the time when people with cancer are often at their lowest ebb.

## 35. *Know your limits*

Before you volunteer your support, ask yourself:

• How much can you reasonably and reliably commit to? Remember that attempting the big gesture, failing and letting a friend down is often worse than not volunteering your services in the first place.

• What else do you have going on in your life? Are you the sort of person who can be relied upon to be there for the long-haul, or better at one-off gestures of support?

• What are you good at? Identify your skills. Can you cook, clean or drive? Are you a whizz on the internet? Do you have either shorthand or keyboard skills, legal or medical/scientific expertise?

• Are you better at doing or organising?

Rather than feeling that you have to 'drop everything' to care for your friend or relative, offer what you can when you can. And instead of taking on more than you can manage, and then disappointing your friend when the enthusiasm wanes, why not try organising a rota? Developing a network of friends to commit bite-sized chunks of time (or money) to help with whatever needs doing – whether it's the ironing or preparing the evening meal or helping out with the school run – helps to spread the load, and can engender a feel-good sense of neighbourliness.

125

## 36. *Be a self-starter. Identify what your friend needs*

Rather than issuing vague 'Let me know what I can do to help' type offers, which give the person with cancer yet one more thing to think about, one more thing to organise, tactfully try to find out where you might most helpfully step in. If you know your friend well, you will probably know what will be most appreciated. If unsure, try to identify what is weighing on them most heavily: it may be the unmown lawn, or the ever-growing pile of ironing, or the homework that needs supervising, or the dog that needs walking, or the evening meal that needs shopping for and preparing, or help with issues over finances or employment rights.

*I was so exhausted by the treatment, I didn't have a spare ounce of energy to do anything, let alone organise a cleaner. The house would have quickly descended into chaos if my friends hadn't taken it upon themselves to step in.* Dee Dee Hope

*It's a question of tuning into one's friend's needs, rather than their cancer, and being guided by what's most important to them – and always has been. Their personality doesn't change as a result of having this disease, and neither do the things that give them comfort. All my instincts are to be very practical. If a sense of order is important to them, I will clean out the fridge and do the washing-up and empty the rubbish. If they don't mind that their house is a mess but have always loved luxury, I will buy wonderful bath oils and scented candles.* Tessa Jowell

*If you know what to do, get on and do it, easily and with no fuss. You help by not fussing around, by just taking it on and, for heaven's sake, by not asking how it should be done.* Mo Mowlam

*Four helpful things to do when around a friend who has been diagnosed with cancer.*
*1. Drop a note*
*2. Make a specific offer of help*
*3. State days and times when you are available*
*4. Wait to hear*
*Fail to honour these four simple rules and you are The Weakest Link. Goodbye.* Anne Robinson

*What was wonderful? People making soup or coming up with new dishes using interesting new flavours, and leaving them quietly on the stove.* Julia Darling

# 37. *Offer to make a list...*

... so that when friends or family who have not read this book

ring or call round and say, 'Is there anything I can do to help?',
your friend can say 'Yes, you might like to do any of the following' and show them the list. It could also help if you take it upon
yourself to ring half a dozen of your friend's better friends and
read the list to them, so they can volunteer to help in whatever
way appeals, and you can tick items off as appropriate.

## 38. *Remember: cancer affects the whole family*

Very often the best way of helping can be by supporting the
other family members. Whisking children away on fun outings
or for special treats, taking spouses out to the movies or the
pub, lightening the load at work… all of these will be gratefully received, coming as they do at a time when principal carers are
likely to be neglecting their own needs.

*Once treatment begins, the support of a network of friends can be
crucial to the whole family. The husband, wife or partner may literally forget to eat, or exist on a diet of hamburgers or fish and
chips. The children can try to protect their parents from pain by not
asking the questions they need answered. Often it's easier for young
people to ask someone else in the family or friendship circle. At
ChildLine I spoke to a teenager who had just learned that her*

*mother had terminal cancer, blamed herself (as children often do), but couldn't tell her mother that the plans the family had made for her were not what she wanted. I encouraged her to speak to her aunt, the child was reassured, and the plans were changed to every-one's benefit.* Esther Rantzen

## 39. *Present yourself as the housework/ laundry/garden/chauffeur fairy*

Either offer your services as a one-off wonder or, better, on an ongoing basis. Commit to a specific time on a specific day. But make sure that you are going to be able to manage it three, six or even 12 months hence, and ring-fence it in your diary so that your friend knows you can be relied upon. If this is difficult for you because you are busy at work all day, how about paying for a cleaner or a gardener to turn up for half a day each week to help out with whatever needs doing?

*Keeping the housework up to Liddy's exacting standards was a source of some stress, especially when anticipating her return home from hospital. So many things needed to be done in preparation for her return that the offer of an extra pair of hands was always welcome. I recall two friends riding on horseback past the window of my office, which is next to the house. A brief word had them parking the horses and putting on the Marigolds! They carried*

*out a wonderful spring-clean and returned later with flowers.*
Peter Gwilliam

> **GROUND RULES** No thanks required; no chats and cups of
> tea unless specifically invited in; a replacement to be found by
> you on days you cannot honour the arrangement; no signs left
> of your presence. Like the Tooth Fairy discreetly leaving a glit-
> tering coin beneath the pillow, your aim is to slip soundlessly
> in and out (if your friend can be persuaded to part with a
> house key, so much the better) leaving, as the only clue to your
> presence, the clean fridge, the pile of freshly ironed clothes in
> the airing cupboard, the meal ready to stick in the oven, the
> dead-headed daffodils and freshly weeded flowerbed, the
> worn-out doggy in his basket (all mud brushed off).

# 40. *Set up a supper rota*

Organise a team of friends to help you, so that everyone com-
mits to cook supper on a specific day once a fortnight or once
a month. This is especially wonderful if treatment turns out to
be so debilitating that even thinking about putting a meal on
the table induces an immediate surge of nausea. I was very fortunate in having a super-organised friend, Demelza Short, three
doors down from us in the terrace where we live in north
London. Within days of my diagnosis, she had rallied a dozen

130

other friends (some of whom I had met only a few times) to cook a weekday evening meal for the family. It worked beautifully, and within a month there were 18 'Colander Girls' (as I called them). An organisational headache was removed, enabling me to devote my depleted energies to the children and their homework. The children loved the surprise packages that arrived at the door, like the 'Secret Santa' game that my daughter played at her school.

> **IMPORTANT** Be sure first to make a list with your friend of what meals will go down well – especially if there are children, who generally have marked likes and dislikes and much prefer plain food. Also ask for guidance about permitted foods if your friend is following a special diet. Many alternative cancer regimens outlaw sugar, dairy, meat and acid-forming foods.

> **GOOD IDEA** Remove a second organisational headache by leaving food in disposable foil dishes so there is no need to return bowls and dishes, nor to remember whose is whose.

# 41. *Hamsters need feeding, too!*

As long as they are fed and watered, and their litter-tray/cages are kept clean, cats and caged creatures do not need a great deal of attention. But dogs and horses often demand a much higher level of care. Taking on 100 per cent responsibility for such animals if your friend is in hospital and there is no one else at home will remove a huge burden at a single stroke. If house-sitting for an extended length of time is impractical, why not organise a rota with a few other friends and take it in turns?

*People forget about the pets. They worry about the person or the children. But when my mother was in hospital, the dogs were her chief concern. We children were grown-up, so she didn't have to worry about us, but she was passionate about her two basset hounds. In fact, she would often say that she preferred dogs to people! Because my father was also being treated for cancer at the same time in a different hospital, neither of them was at home to look after the dogs, and to begin with it preyed on her mind, so the friends who volunteered to come in twice a day to feed and walk them took on the status of real heroes in her eyes.* Gaby Roslin

## 42. *Set up a group email*

The flurry of calls and enquiries following a diagnosis does not always simmer down. Friends and non-immediate family need to know, urgently, what is happening, what the doctors said, how the clinic appointment went, whether chemo/radiotherapy/surgery is scheduled this week/next week or any time soon. As the questions come thick and fast, it is all too easy for the person at the centre of this well-intentioned curiosity to feel like the Ancient Mariner, compelled to repeat his story for eternity.

When a great friend of mine, Liddy Oldroyd, was diagnosed with a carcinoid tumour that had spread to her liver, her husband would email a group of 80 of her closest friends (she was pathologically gregarious) with details of her hospital admissions and visiting hours, at one point linking us up to a medical website that explained (in colour!) the complex surgical chemo-embolisation procedure that she was about to undergo in such detail that we felt as knowledgeable as if we'd been personally briefed by her consultant. Thus genned up, we did not need to bombard the family with calls, nor to drain her energies with irritating questions on our visits, which were then reserved for more enjoyable personal exchanges.

**HOW TO SET UP A GROUP EMAIL** (using Microsoft Outlook Express)

**To create a group of contacts (Group)**

**1.** In the **Address Book**, select the folder in which you want to create a Group. Click **New** on the toolbar, and then click **New Group**.

**2.** The **Properties** dialog box opens. In the **Group Name** box, choose and then type the name of the group.

**3.** There are several ways to add people to the group:

a) To add a person from your **Address Book** list, click **Select Members**, and then click a name from the **Address Book**

133

list in the left-hand column. Click **Select** in the right-hand column and then click **OK** at the bottom.

b) To add a person directly to the group without adding the name to your **Address Book**, repeat a) above and then type the person's name and email address in the lower half of the **Properties** dialog box, and then click **Add**.

c) To add a person to both the group and your **Address Book**, click **New Contact** and fill in the appropriate information.

**4.** Repeat for each addition until your group is defined.

**To send emails to Group list**

**1.** On the toolbar, click the **Create Mail** button.

**2.** In the **To** or **Cc** or **Bcc** boxes, type the email name of the group. Use the **Bcc** (blind copy) box to ensure confidentiality, by hiding names and email addresses of recipients.

**3.** Select **All Headers** on the **View** menu.

**4.** In the **Subject** box, type a message title.

**5.** Type your message, and then click **Send** on the toolbar.

# 43. *Offer to set up a blog...*

A 'web-log', or internet diary, can update everyone instantly on any new development at the click of a mouse, wherever they are in the world. It takes minutes to set up, costs nothing and has the great advantage that, rather than swallowing up more time and precious energy, new well-wishers can be directed to a web address to mainline as much information as they want.

I set up a blog about three weeks after my diagnosis. The constantly ringing telephone was sending us mad ('It's the f****** phone again,' my 14-year-old daughter would say with weary alliteration), but I recognised that certain calls had to be taken and visits received, especially from those geographically furthest from the epicentre; because they were not able to 'pop in' to see me and catch up on the latest developments, far-flung friends were particularly prey to the very worst fears and imaginings. And then it suddenly came to me. Why not take advantage of the world wide web to keep everyone informed at the click of a mouse, in whatever remote corner of the globe they happened to be?

From its inception, my blog has epitomised the true meaning of 'interactive'. Friends and family can visit the site to find out what I'm up to, how I'm feeling and how the family is doing; while I can log on to enjoy their comments and observations and to feel a little less alone. We even have quizzes and competitions and a regular race to be the first to post a comment. What's more, the time it takes to post a new entry, usually less than an hour, is more than offset by the time saved answering calls and enquiries, however well meant. These days, the phone rings even less than it used to before my diagnosis, and I am also spared endless energy-sapping repetition. For example, I recently met a friend I hadn't seen since I found out

I had cancer. Because she had been closely following the blog and was therefore fully up to speed, we were able to pick up in the here and now, without wasting precious time backtracking over recent grim events, which would have cast a dark cloud over our meeting.

*When my mother was diagnosed with lung cancer last year, she set up a website on which she now keeps a diary so that anyone, at any time, can see how she is. This diary not only really helps me, as I am away at boarding school and often cannot face the hourly minimum phone call home, but also keeps the phone from ringing 24 hours a day with well-wishers after an update. People make comments after each entry and there is now an entire community of friends and family who contribute to the blog, which not only informs people how my mother is coping but also inspires all those who are a part of it.* Archie Stebbings (aged 17)

### HOW TO SET UP A BLOG

Select your web host: click on www.lights.com/weblogs/hosting.html for a large list of blogging services with brief descriptions. Three of the biggest players in the field are www.blogger.com – free, easy to use, run by Google, but it doesn't offer image hosting (ie, it won't allow you to upload images directly to the same site as your written content); www.livejournal.com – two levels of service, free or paid, and offers image hosting; and www.spaces.msn.com – run by

Microsoft, free service allows you to post images and works in conjunction with a hotmail account or MSN passport for easy sign-in.

Once you have chosen your host site, follow the simple steps and, in less than half a dozen clicks, you'll be away.

## *... and volunteer to post the entries on your friend's behalf*

You can do this either by taking down the gist of what they want to say and expanding it into readable form, or by taking down the details verbatim and then transcribing them.

## 44. *If you are money-rich but time-poor, consider clubbing together to buy in extra help*

When needs are considerable and finances a problem, a group of better-off friends might consider clubbing together to hire a daily help or housekeeper or nanny on a part-time or full-time basis as the need, and money available, dictates. Divided by a reasonable number, the cost per head can be very manageable – almost invisible, in fact. And it's lovely to know that, in the absence of hands-on help, you are able to do something that is making a real difference on a daily basis.

When an old university friend first became ill, about a year after being diagnosed with liver cancer, she had three young children – aged 14, 12 and seven – and a long line of unsatisfactory, non-driving, non-fluent-English-speaking au pairs. The strain of trying to orchestrate the childcare during her increasing stays in hospital was telling on the family and absorbing large amounts of her husband's time which would have been much better spent as the family's breadwinner.

Insightfully identifying the need, her two best friends took it upon themselves to rope in a large group of about 20 of us, and asked us to commit a small amount of money every month, up front, by direct debit, to pay for a nanny/housekeeper: a luxury that was beyond the personal financial reach of two self-employed people, one now not working at all. They advertised and interviewed and, together with my friend and her husband, found the perfect person: a practical, middle-aged antipodean.

All we did was shell out a smallish amount of money every month that, for working men and women with reasonable incomes, made no noticeable dent on our own standard of living. But the impact on the family's quality of life was dramatic. The school runs, the weekly shop, the dog's walking schedule, the evening meals and the relative chaos into which the house had descended were sorted.

# 45. *Offer to find out about grants and entitlements*

Cancer can be impoverishing. In a survey carried out by CancerBACUP, nearly two-thirds of the respondents said they had experienced financial difficulties after their cancer treatment, so it's hardly surprising that anxiety about money is cited second only to physical pain as the major cause of stress for those of us living with cancer and our families.

If we are working and have to cease for a considerable stretch of time, we can suffer a significant loss of income – at the same time as incurring a raft of additional costs associated with the illness (travelling to the hospital, parking, prescription charges, heating the home all day every day). Single people, who are solely responsible for the running of their home, may be under particular financial pressure.

Many cancer patients do not get the financial help that they are entitled to. In 2003, Macmillan Cancer Relief's report *The Unclaimed Millions* revealed that a total of £126 million from just two state benefits (Disability Living Allowance and Attendance Allowance) was going unclaimed by thousands of terminally ill cancer patients in the UK. Don't let your friend be one of them.

Depending on the stage of cancer, your friend may be eligible for one or more of the following state benefits:

- Disability Living Allowance (not means-tested and currently just over £100 a week, which can usually be back-dated to the time of diagnosis)
- Attendance Allowance
- Incapacity Benefit
- Carer's Allowance
- Housing and Council Tax Benefit
- Income Support, including disability and carer premiums
- Working Tax Credit
- Child Tax Credit
- Council Tax Rebate
- Help from the Social Fund

Most cancer centres, based in the larger hospitals, have people on hand to give expert advice on everything from financial entitlements to welfare and employment rights. Ask your clinical nurse specialist to book an appointment.

The Macmillan Benefits Helpline (0808 801 0304, Monday to Friday, 10am to 5pm, or Wednesdays, 12 noon to 5pm) is a new telephone advice service for people in the UK with cancer, and for their families and carers, who need help to access benefits and other kinds of financial support. Calls to the helpline are answered by experienced advisers who can check exactly the benefits and other kinds of financial help to which people are entitled. They can also help to fill in the necessary forms and make a claim. Alternatively, find out about grants and/or benefits that may be available by phoning the Macmillan CancerLine (freephone 0800 808 2020) and asking for the booklet *What Can I Claim?*, or call the Benefit Enquiry Line (0800 882 200) or your local Welfare Rights Unit (phone your local authority).

People with cancer can also apply to Macmillan for a small grant to help meet specific costs arising from having cancer, such as fuel and travel. Last year, grants totalling more than £6.5 million were made to over 17,000 people, most of which were sent out within three days of application. Call the Macmillan CancerLine to see if your friend is eligible, and complete an application on their behalf.

*Having cancer places enormous strains on your marriage, your family and your bank balance.* Sally Hamilton

**NB** Depending on the stage of your friend's cancer, and the degree to which their mobility is compromised, they may also be entitled to exemption of road tax and a disabled (blue) badge, which can take some of the pressure out of parking when attending hospital appointments. Help with transport to and from clinic appointments and chemo/radiotherapy sessions is often available: check with hospital staff.

If they are being treated in a hospital in central London, and drive or are being driven through the congestion zone, they can have the charge reimbursed by the hospital, which will in turn be reimbursed by Transport for London. As their companion, you can make practical use of waiting time by filling in forms, etc.

Other forms of help with transport are also available. Explore the Dial-a-Ride scheme, which offers a door-to-door service for people who are not able to use public transport. You may have to fill in an application form for the doctor to sign. Find the number in your phone book, under Dial- (or, occasionally, Ring-) a-Ride. The service cannot be used for hospital visits, but can be used for social trips, going to the hairdressers, and so on. Journeys need to be booked in advance and are charged at a public transport rate.

If finances are a problem, it may be possible to obtain help towards the cost of a holiday from a cancer charity. Find out more about this from health professionals.

If special provisions have had to be made in the home as a result of cancer, your friend may be entitled to a reduction in council tax.

# 46. *Ask about deferring payment of unavoidable bills and charges*

Make a list with your friend of the bills that are piling up – the rent or mortgage, council tax, heating and electricity. And then pick up the phone. With your friend's blessing, contact the manager of the bank or building society that arranged the mortgage to explain the situation and ask if they would be prepared to suspend payments for a few months on receipt of a letter from the hospital consultant or social worker. (You could ring the clinical nurse specialist at the hospital and ask her to organise this and then make several photocopies.)

Alternatively, it may be possible to extend the term of the mortgage, so your friend has less to pay each month, or the bank or building society may agree to accept interest-only payments. Help with interest payments may be available from the Department for Work and Pensions. Ring the local council office about deferring council tax payments, the landlord about rental payments and the providers of utilities such as water, gas, electricity and telephone if your friend anticipates difficulty in meeting payment dates for these services.

# 47. *Help to sort out travel insurance*

Arranging insurance is notoriously difficult, and often deeply upsetting, for anyone with a potentially life-threatening condition, particularly cancer, as it doesn't take long to discover that PWC (People With Cancer) are the pariahs of the human race. A dispiriting series of calls with a succession of brokers trying to find someone – anyone – to provide cover for a fortnight in

Spain, and then trying to summon the funds to pay the premium, is enough to take the gloss off the prospect of any holiday.

If your friend has until now had an annually renewed travel insurance policy, there is still an obligation to notify the insurers of any change in medical circumstance, and the insurers can then decide to exempt that condition from the cover offered, even if the year's policy still has some way to go. It is then incumbent upon your friend to find someone who will insure them for what is known as a 'pre-existing medical condition'.

There are some companies that specialise in providing such cover. They may carry out a medical screening over the phone, using a questionnaire to score responses and so assess the degree of risk, and thereby the premium. If the condition is more serious, they may require confirmation from medical personnel that your friend is fit to fly and travel at all.

Some of the questions can be seriously intrusive. I was asked point-blank if my condition was terminal, and when I confirmed that, indeed, it was, I was then asked how long I had been given (a figure I never asked for and never wanted), and was then warned that I was almost certainly 'too great a risk' to be insured anyway! Having had someone on hand to make these calls for me, and spare me such a brutal inquisition, would have been a blessing.

**INSURANCE TIPS** Offer to ring round to compare quotes and costs on your friend's behalf, having made a list of the basic details of your friend's cancer (type, stage, date of diagnosis, treatment undergone, medication). The following companies claim to specialise in offering travel insurance to people with cancer, at a considerable premium: Freedom Travel Insurance (0870 774 3760); All Clear (0870 777 9339); FreeSpirit (0845 230 5000); MediCover (0870 735 3600); Medi Travelcover 01252 782392 (best for advanced cancer, but reserves the right to choose and refuse).

# 48. *Offer to find out about sick pay*

The world of sick pay and benefits is a jungle; being on hand to unravel some of the threads will be much appreciated.

All employees who earn enough to pay National Insurance (NI) are eligible for Statutory Sick Pay (SSP) for a maximum of 28 weeks. Self-employed people who have made regular NI contributions are eligible for Incapacity Benefit. If your friend is still unable to work after that time, they may be able to claim Incapacity Benefit, via Form SSP1 from the Department for Work and Pensions.

They may also be entitled to Occupational Sick Pay. This will be detailed in their contract of employment. This is usually paid as a top-up to SSP – they won't get both, but SSP becomes part of their Occupational Sick Pay. People who are not eligible for SSP/Incapacity Benefit can apply for Income Support.

145

Your friend can keep claiming some benefits even after returning to work, such as Disability Living Allowance, but others such as Incapacity Benefit may be affected.

For further information, ring the Benefit Enquiry Line on 0800 882 200.

**REMEMBER!** A sick note from the GP will be necessary to claim a benefit. A medical test may sometimes also be required.

*My friend is about to start chemo for lung cancer. His greatest worry is whether he will be able to keep up with all the paperwork, or if the business will go belly-up. He daren't risk people knowing how ill he is.* Kenny Potter

*I was so lucky. I had complete support from everybody at work, with my colleagues helping to take the pressure off at every turn. I did feel a bit guilty that I was not able to be there yet was still being paid, especially after seeing how the financial burden of being off work can pile on the stress and how unsympathetic some work places can be… I know of people who have had to go back to work before being fit or ready to and it's taken them much longer to recover.* Vicky Baglioni

*I was lucky. My boss was fantastically accommodating. She kept my job open for me all the way through my sick leave. I was paid a mixture of full-pay, half-pay and Statutory Sick Pay. And*

*when I went back, I was able to build my hours up gradually.*
Dee Dee Hope

# 49. *Put them in the picture about their rights at work*

Ninety thousand people of working age are diagnosed with cancer every year, and according to the latest statistics nearly a third are deterred from rejoining the workforce once their treatment is over. This is not because of the severity of their cancer, but because they get no support in the way of practical work-adjustment policies or flexible working arrangements that might allow a phased return to work – even though they may have every right to expect certain concessions from their employers, following a recent amendment to the Disability Discrimination Act 1995. Working people diagnosed with cancer are entitled to:

1. Not tell their employers that they are having tests for cancer.

2. Expect their employers to make certain changes to working hours and practices to help them if they wish to continue work.

3. Challenge their dismissal as unfair if they are dismissed

because of their illness, even if they work only part-time.

Most employers will hold a job open if an employee is having treatment for cancer, but it may depend on the particular contract of employment.

Under the latest amendment to the Disability Discrimination Act, people with cancer who have, or have had, symptoms that have an adverse effect on their normal day-to-day activities have certain rights, which include the expectation that the employer will make 'reasonable adjustments' to workplaces and working practices. Such adjustments may include:

- Allowing time off to attend medical appointments
- Modifying a job description to take away tasks that cause particular difficulty
- Allowing some flexibility in working hours
- Allowing extra breaks to cope with fatigue
- Temporarily restricting the employee to 'light duties'
- Moving the employee to a post with more suitable duties (with the employee's agreement)
- Providing appropriate washroom facilities
- Allowing working from home
- Allowing a gradual return to work

Research by CancerBACUP has shown that people not offered information by their employers about managing work issues are four times more likely to find that their working lives have deteriorated as a result of their illness, while those not offered flexible or alternative working arrangements are 15 times more likely to experience significant financial difficulties. Urge your friend to arrange a meeting with their employer, human resources department or occupational health staff before returning to work to discuss any changes that could be implemented to facilitate their re-entry to the workplace, such as a phased return, whereby they gradually increase the hours worked and slowly ease themselves back into office life.

If your friend is covered by the terms of the Disability Discrimination Act and feels discriminated against by an employer, seek advice from the Disability Rights Commission, whose website (www.drc-gb.org) gives comprehensive information on employment rights and also runs an online advice service; alternatively, call 08457 622 633.

If cancer causes disability that affects the kind of work done, your friend may be eligible for help from a scheme called Access to Work – find out more from the Department for Work and Pensions website (www.dwp.gov.uk).

## … for both of you

If you are the partner or parent of someone having cancer treatment and you need to take time off work to accompany them to hospital appointments and/or look after them, you may be entitled to take compassionate leave, dependency leave or unpaid leave.

Under the Employment Rights Act 1996, employees have a statutory right to time off for dependants. A 'dependant' is someone you have responsibility for, such as a child or an elderly parent. A parent of a child with cancer is entitled to up to 18 weeks of unpaid leave. Some employers may allow paid leave to be taken, while others allow longer than the official entitlement. Guidance leaflets can be found at www.dti.gov.uk/er/timeoff.htm.

Some family members of people with cancer may experience discrimination should they wish to take time off. As family members are not covered by the Disability Discrimination Act, there is less legal protection; get advice from your local Citizens Advice Bureau.

# Searching...

A diagnosis of cancer is often accompanied by a disconcerting sense of losing all control. No sooner has the news been broken than we are swept at dizzying speed on to the one-size-fits-all conveyor belt that prevails in many over-stretched hospitals and oncology departments. No longer a person any more, but a patient or, worse, a cancer: 'the melanoma in bed 4'. No wonder so many of us, desperate to regain a measure of control, find ourselves drawn to therapies that offer a more personal approach: time to talk, a higher degree of hope than can be found in the more measured mainstream, and an accent on the whole person (psychological, emotional and spiritual as well as physical) rather than the illness. In conversations with other people with cancer, adjectives such as 'empowering' came up again and again in relation to alternative and complementary therapies, but were noticeably absent in descriptions of conventional medicine, however successful.

*I was in a dilemma about whether to go ahead with chemo: could I take it? I remember sitting in my workroom, with the warm autumn sun pouring through the window, and I suddenly had a huge surge of energy and a feeling almost of excitement and adventure. I decided that I would go through the lot, plus all the alternative therapies I could find, plus eating really well.* Mary MacCarthy

*I found taking control of my situation helped me feel that I was the one making the decisions (although I wasn't). It is very easy to feel swept along by all the medics, and I hated feeling that there was nothing else I could do. A specialist diet, no alcohol or dairy products, was my way of saying, 'I am doing everything I can to help myself and I am the one in control.' A great friend who runs an organic delivery business sent us a box of vegetables and fruit every week as his present to us.* Georgie Hall

*Even if I wasn't doing all these things for myself, I would be doing*

152

*them for the children, who have been so very frightened, and real-*
*ly need to know not only that I am doing everything I can to save*
*my life, but that they can play a part in this endeavour too. On*
*some days, it feels like we are all united in one gigantic family mis-*
*sion. They love bringing me my cups of green tea, or counting out*
*my vitamin pills, or reminding me to take the half-dozen Brazil*
*nuts that constitute my daily selenium dose, or sitting with me*
*while I play my visualisation and relaxation tapes.* Dee Dee Hope

The truth is that wherever you stand on the conventional/
alternative continuum, things look very different the other side
of a cancer diagnosis. Believe me. Before my diagnosis, I was by
profession a sceptic. Unlike many other glossy-magazine jour-
nalists, I eschewed the fashionable mania for all things New
Agey, being suspicious to a point of total dismissiveness about
quack cures. Their breathless testimonials of miraculous remis-
sions and doctor-defying recoveries were, I was quite convinced, just a short step away from believing in little green men
from Mars. Then I was diagnosed with stage IV cancer, treated
with the utmost care and concern by my medical team, but
offered little in the way of hope, and suddenly, as I wrote in a
feature on my changed perspectives for *Vogue* magazine, I found
the landscape had changed utterly.

*BC – before my cancer – I prided myself on being able to sniff out*
*a charlatan at a hundred paces. I was a founder member of the*

*Campaign Against Health Fraud. Press releases proclaiming the powers of wacky remedies were consigned to the bin faster than you could say 'bullshit'. In those days, I was convinced that I was protecting my readers from cruel rip-offs preying on the hopes and fears of desperate, vulnerable, sick people. Now I am a desperate, vulnerable, sick person myself, however, I am beginning to find myself strangely drawn to stories of people who were 'given' three months to live, swallowed shark's fin cartilage and went on to celebrate silver wedding anniversaries and outlive all their contemporaries.*

*AD – after my diagnosis – my bathroom shelves bear witness to my new mindset. I now swallow 40 different pills and potions every day, from high-potency vitamins and immune boosters to a controversial ayurvedic remedy called carctol (which comes with a hard-to-follow alkaline diet and the imperative to drink three litres of water a day), and a mysterious agaricus mushroom extract specially couriered over from the rainforests of Brazil.* Deborah Hutton, *Vogue*, July 2005

At its simplest, the quest for alternative or complementary approaches involves self-help measures and/or fairly well-accepted therapies that boost energy, enhance well-being and make us better able to withstand the side-effects of conventional treatment. There is a good body of research, for example, demonstrating that acupuncture can be very helpful in reducing the nausea and vomiting associated with some kinds of chemotherapy. 'There's now enough rational evidence of the benefits of therapies such as reflexology and acupuncture to call these approaches supportive rather than alternative or even complementary,' says Andrew Anderson, head of the Maggie's Centre in Edinburgh. 'And to get away from the sandals-and-lentils image that does so much to put so many people off.'

At the far end of the continuum, however, lie the much more controversial, much more radical, truly alternative treatments which demand that their adherents turn their backs on what their doctors advise, swapping conventional care for programmes of rigorous diet, supplements and injections of anything from mistletoe to pancreatic enzymes.

While doctors are increasingly open to their patients using complementary therapies alongside mainstream medicine – half of all GP practices in England now provide access to these supportive therapies in some way, and one in three makes acupuncture available to their patients – they are likely to be less enthusiastic if patients plan to use them in place of it. While most doctors don't believe that there is valid evidence that any alternative approach can cure cancer or slow its growth, the alternative therapists often put such a seductive spin on what they are offering that it can seem (especially to those, like me, with very poor prognoses) an irresistible antidote to the gloomy pessimism that rules in the nation's cancer clinics.

Back in the 1950s, for example, Max Gerson, founder of the controversial Gerson diet (which involves drinking freshly prepared organic vegetable juice, along with a number of supplements and self-administered injections, including thyroid hormones and liver extracts), claimed a 30 per cent response rate, even with people who were terminally ill. Although the few small studies to put his diet to the test have found no evidence to support this, people continue to find it difficult to turn their backs on anything claiming to hold hope of remission when they have in effect been written off as no-hopers by their regular clinicians, as evidenced by the enduring popularity of his extraordinarily demanding diet.

*Where most medical-scientific information is either inconclusive or honestly negative, most alternative 'information' is anecdotal and unrelentingly positive. Reading alternative literature, you begin to get the giddy feeling that everybody treated by orthodox medicine dies, and everybody treated by alternative medicine lives (except those who were first treated by orthodox methods: they all die).*

*We began an intensive investigation of virtually every type of alternative treatment available: macrobiotics, Gerson diet, Kelley enzymes, Burton, Burzynski, psychic surgery, faith healing, Livingston-Wheeler, Hoxsey, laetrile, megavitamins, immunotherapy, visualisation, acupuncture, affirmations, and so on... Although we were both great fans of alternative and holistic medicine, careful scrutiny showed that none of the alternatives had any substantial success against grade-four tumors. These tumors are the Nazis of the cancer crowd, and they are not terribly impressed*

*with wheatgrass juice and sweet thoughts. You have to nuke these*
*bastards if you are going to have any chance at all – and that's where*
*white man's medicine comes in.* Ken Wilber, *Grace and Grit*

> **DID YOU KNOW?** The first Europe-wide survey on the use
> of complementary and alternative medical approaches, pub-
> lished in *Annals of Oncology* in early 2005, found that a third
> of cancer patients in Europe were using these approaches, with
> users tending to be female, younger, better educated and to
> have cancers with poorer prognoses.

# 50. *Take your lead from your friend – do not force your personal health ideologies on them*

Should you help friends by pointing them in the direction of an
alternative/complementary therapist, or by sending them one
of the hundreds of books on offer with upbeat titles such as
*Sharks Don't Get Cancer*? Lots of the people I spoke to still shudder at the memory of being swamped by well-meaning but
unwanted letters offering to put them in touch with assorted
dowsers and pendulum swingers, crystal healers and inter-
preters of tea leaves and ley lines who had sent their best friend's
cousin's incurable cancer into miraculous, indefinite remission.

*As soon as word got out, I started getting letters on gritty recycled paper from old friends in Glastonbury who wanted to introduce me to healers and homeopaths and herbalists, and I turned them all down. There is not a scrap of evidence that alternative or complementary medicine does any good at all apart from cheering you up, and I had my own ways of doing that. I also resent the implication which lies beneath complementary approaches that a disease is always your own fault. You ate the wrong food, lived the wrong lifestyle or thought the wrong kind of thoughts.* Martyn Harris, 'This is not the time to die', *The Spectator*, 19 August 1995*

*The really unhelpful people were those who insisted on giving me books on alternative therapies I personally didn't want. I wasn't into thinking my cancer away; I didn't want the Bristol approach. I counted 15 and threw them all away.* Dr Ann McPherson

The message has to be: don't superimpose your own agenda. Complementary therapies can be very time-consuming and very expensive – especially if, like me, you are following several different approaches – and they demand a high level of commitment. Not only can you quickly find your life ruled by the imperative to do your visualisation and your yoga and your breathing exercises, while boiling up your Chinese herbs, juicing your organic vegetables and swallowing dozens of vitamin and nutritional supplements a day – and that's in between the acupuncture/nutritionist/intravenous vitamin infusion appointments – but the sweeping lifestyle changes they demand can place an impossible load on an already weakened system.

As a rule, the more they promise, the more these approaches demand in the way of energy, input and commitment: go organic, they instruct, have all your fillings replaced, juice your own vegetables on the hour every hour, squeezing in four coffee enemas for good measure, substitute all your household cleaning products for less 'toxic' alternatives, avoid dairy products, fatty foods, all sugars (this when many of us are battling not to lose any more weight). Oh yes, and do all this while avoiding all stress! As though trying to change the habits of a lifetime were not stressful at the best of times, let alone when ill and weak and shocked and vulnerable.

*I had so little energy, I decided I didn't want to use it up juicing and sprouting. I wanted life to be as normal as it could be, I wanted to be with the family, sharing their meals, not shut away giving myself coffee enemas. I did concentrate on eating good-quality food, drinking herb teas and having weekly massages, however. It meant a lot to have a smiley, sunny person do this wonderful thing that made me feel very good, and it helped to relieve all those little aches and pains.* Heidi Locher

Recognise that it can take a lot to summon the strength to turn down these offers. So be tactful. Do not impose and do not insist. If you do feel you have the name of a helpful therapy/therapist, send a card or an email giving details and asking them to contact you if they are interested in finding out more; write that you will otherwise assume they are not – this small but vital addition removes even the need for a reply.

## 51. *If your friend is receptive to alternative approaches, consider a relevant gift...*

### An inspirational book

*A Time to Heal* by Beata Bishop – a triumphal recovery story by a graduate of the controversial Gerson diet: vegetable juices, liver extracts, coffee enemas, the lot.

*The Bristol Approach to Living with Cancer* by Helen Cooke – a good introduction to supportive complementary approaches as offered by the renowned Bristol Cancer Help Centre.

*Getting Well Again* by Carl and Stephanie Simonton – visualisation and meditation techniques.

*Living Proof: a medical mutiny* by Michael Gearin-Tosh – the personal story of one man's miraculous remission of the multiple myeloma he was told would kill him in months.

*Love, Medicine and Miracles* by Bernie Siegel – traces the experiences of what Siegal calls 'exceptional patients' and gives guidelines to help readers become one themselves.

*Your Life in Your Hands* by Jane Plant – a non-dairy diet book written by a professor of medicine for people with breast cancer.

*Cancer as a Turning Point* by Lawrence LeShan – out of print, but available via Amazon (www.amazon.co.uk), this cult book helps people with cancer to find meaning, and healing, through the living out of unrealised dreams.

**A session with a registered therapist to restore a sense of being in control, and enhance well-being**
Consider a session of acupuncture or reiki or spiritual healing, an aromatherapy massage, Alexander Technique lesson or relaxation class.

**If money is no object, a residential weekend away**
Bristol Cancer Help Centre runs two- and five-day courses, teaching practical skills in the form of a range of self-help techniques such as meditation and visualisation (call 0117 980 1502 or book online at www.bristolcancerhelp.org).

**If chemotherapy is on the cards, supportive homeopathic remedies**
Ring a leading homeopathic chemists such as Ainsworths (020 7935 5330) and tell them what drug regime your friend will be on, and get them to post specific remedies to help support them through it.

> **NB** Always seek a qualified therapist who belongs to a professional body, rather than risk ending up in the hands of some plausible charlatan who learnt his trade in a couple of weekend workshops in Bognor Regis. Not only does it guarantee a certain level of training and code of professional conduct, but it will also provide a forum for complaint in the event of malpractice. Standards of training vary hugely both from therapy to therapy and within each of the professions, from the osteopaths and chiropractors who are regulated by law, like doctors, all the way down to people qualifying by correspondence course, with no hands-on experience required.
>
> Find information on each therapy and how to access properly trained practitioners for all the leading types of complementary therapy by downloading *Complementary Healthcare: a guide for patients* on the Foundation for Integrated Health's website (www.ifhealth.org.uk) or call the foundation on 020 7619 6140.

## ... and check out what's available on the NHS

An increasing number of cancer treatment centres offer a limited range of therapies such as psychotherapy, counselling, massage and meditation. And a few may also offer aromatherapy, reflexology, acupuncture, iscador (extract of mistletoe given by injection or oral drops), hypnotherapy, healing, visualisation and art therapy, so it's always worth asking the hospital/clinical nurse specialist what might be available.

**DID YOU KNOW?** Homeopathy is available on the NHS and has been since its inception in 1949. There are five homeopathic hospitals offering a complementary cancer care programme that can be used alongside regular hospital treatment in Bristol, Glasgow, Liverpool, London and Tunbridge Wells. Ask an oncologist, consultant or GP for a referral.

## 52. Help your friend to avoid being exploited

When I was first diagnosed, I went to see a range of nutritionally minded alternative therapists. Some were very good and responsible, giving me practical, balanced advice that would help support the mainstream treatment I was undergoing. Others ranted for hours about the deficiencies of the 'slash, poison and burn' orthodox medical approach and sent me away for rafts of diagnostic tests that would have set me back more than £1,000 at clinics that showed much more interest in the expiry date on my credit card than in extending any possible expiry date of my own.

*I am president of HealthWatch, an organisation that promotes evidence-based treatments and is sceptical of some orthodox medicine, let alone unproven 'complementary' approaches. There are some bad doctors and some very sensitive and caring unconventional 'therapists', but in my experience alternative therapies are generally no better than placebo [fake treatments] and an intellectual fraud. After all, they would be conventional treatments if they really worked. There is no giant conspiracy among doctors to allow us to suffer unnecessarily; the regulators are not perverse to demand that pharmaceutical companies have to prove their products are effective and safe; there is no credible economic incentive for conventional markets to marginalise services and products that could be popular and profitable.*

*I find it patronising that when somebody has a grim prognosis we should treat them as children and encourage them to believe in Father Christmas; even worse that charlatans should prey on people at their most vulnerable. The claims aren't always just white lies; alternative health is a multibillion-pound industry.*

*One person I knew spent hundreds of thousands of pounds that his family would later need in the hope of prolonging his life, and failed. He was not particularly close to me. I have since often asked myself what, had he been closer, I would have done, what I should have done.* Nick Ross

What indeed? I talked to Dr Sosie Kassab, director of complementary cancer services at the Royal London Homeopathic Hospital, who is both a homeopath and a conventionally trained physician, and is therefore in a better position than most to evaluate the benefits and risks of both approaches. How would she support and advise a close friend or family member who was contemplating abandoning conventional therapy and following an alternative path instead?

'I would suggest they try and accept as much conventional medicine as they can,' she replied, 'while exploring all the options they need to explore alongside. If quality of life is suffering, if the advantages of treatment are seeming to be outweighed by the disadvantages, and they are seriously considering turning their back on conventional medicine altogether, I would urge them to get a balanced view by asking their oncologist what can be achieved through the conventional route by way of a) complete cure or b) if there is no prospect of cure, then prolonging survival and c) if there is only a small chance of prolonging survival, then alleviating symptoms and enhancing the quality of life. Once my relative or friend had

165

that information, I would feel they would be much better placed to come to a good decision, and I would respect and attempt to support them in whatever they did.'

*I never thought I would agree to chemotherapy. I was always supremely health-conscious and had tremendous fears about putting any form of toxin into my body, and here I was considering allowing my doctors to poison me within an inch of my life. I also had fears about the long-term effects on my immune system. I resisted it for a long time, but finally decided that, on reflection, despite its side-effects, chemotherapy was my best chance of being cured.* Sally Marshall

## 53. *Volunteer to gather some hard information. Sift the factual from the fictional and even the fraudulent...*

Because unorthodox approaches have such a high level of implausibility, and may even fly in the face of science, the medical profession often dismisses them as not having 'a shred of scientific evidence' to support them. This is not quite true. There are some respectable research studies, some of which show real value, and you can access them via the websites given on the next two pages. It is also the case that research into

166

complementary approaches is very thin on the ground, partly because there is such difficulty getting funding for any treatment that does not offer the prospect of big financial returns, and partly because of the nature of the treatments themselves. While conventional medicine typically uses treatments that can be readily submitted to placebo-controlled double-blind randomised trials (the so-called 'gold standard'), many complementary and alternative treatments have to be tailored to the individual, which makes rigorous clinical trials more difficult.

The reality is that, with genetic research still at too early a stage to tell us reliably who will benefit from a certain treatment and who will not, a lot of conventional medicine is itself based on guesswork and finger-crossing. Any doctor will concede that the whole field of cancer research poses many unknowns, and that our knowledge base is still relatively small compared with most other diseases, which are much better understood.

In his memorable book *Living Proof: a medical mutiny*, Michael Gearin-Tosh, an Oxford don who declined chemotherapy for a serious blood cancer called multiple myeloma and instead went on the controversial Gerson diet, describes how his odyssey for knowledge took him to see an internationally renowned professor of surgery at Oxford University.

*'Do you think I am mad to try what I am doing?' I ask.*

*Sir David Weatherall is a man who thinks for as long as he wishes before he speaks. A minute or two pass. 'What you must understand, Mr Gearin-Tosh, is that we know so little about how the body works.'* Michael Gearin-Tosh, *Living Proof*

Play devil's advocate by logging on to www.quackwatch.org, a forthright fraud-busting site, which examines the claims of all the major alternative therapies (scroll to 'Cancer questionable therapies' for the low-down on a wide range of therapies and so-called 'cancer cures') and almost invariably finds them wanting.

While it's a good counter-balance to all that alternative spin, a more measured view can be gained from the US government's excellent complementary and alternative medicine website (www.nccam.nih.gov), sponsored by the National Institutes for Health, which also includes some useful cautions and tips; and/or the website of the Memorial Sloan-Kettering Cancer Center in New York (www.mskcc.org), the most famous cancer hospital in the world, which has a valuable section on herbal and other unorthodox remedies, complete with references to published trials (enter 'about herbs, botanicals and other products' in the search box and click go). *The British Medical Journal* site has a collection of more than a hundred articles relating to complementary medicine that have been published in the journal since 1998 (http://bmj.bmjjournals.com/collections; click on 'Complementary medicine').

While information from all of the above can be downloaded free, serious site-seekers might consider subscribing to Fact (Focus on Alternative and Complementary Therapies;

www.pharmpress.com/fact). This British-based online magazine runs a systematic search of the world research literature on complementary and alternative medicine, and has a comprehensive database dating back ten years.

## 54. *Signpost the more reputable websites*

The world wide web has transformed access to information of all kinds, and especially information about health. More and more people rely on the internet for information about their own healthcare, some of it very sound and some of it highly misleading. The realm of alternative and complementary medicine is a particular minefield. If you enter 'alternative medicine' on Google, you will be directed to more than 37 million possible websites, many not worth the virtual paper they are written on, and some positively harmful. A survey of websites giving information about complementary medicine for cancer, published in the *Annals of Oncology* in 2004, concluded that 'the most popular websites on complementary and alternative medicine for cancer offer information of extremely variable quality. Many endorse unproven therapies and some are outright dangerous.' You have been warned.

*When my daughter-in-law discovered she had breast cancer, she avidly read everything she could on the internet and, as she is by nature very imaginative and often overcome with foreboding, it fed her emotions in a rather negative way.* Susan Fellowes

So how do you sift the wheat from the chaff? I asked Professor Edzard Ernst, Britain's only professor of complementary medicine, who is based at the Peninsula Medical School at the universities of Exeter and Plymouth. His department has investigated a number of websites and organisations offering advice on complementary and alternative approaches to cancer and has found that the information supplied is often misleading or inaccurate or, worse, that it has the potential to cause harm. Professor Ernst suggests asking yourself the following:

• Is the website commercially motivated? Sites with something to sell are generally the most inaccurate and potentially hazardous. If you are being pressed to purchase a product, be cautious. At best, it may only harm your bank balance. At worst, a product may either be toxic or cause harm because it aims to replace effective medical treatments.

• Who owns the website? Is it clear? Is it sponsored by government, or run by a hospital or university or reputable medical or health-based association? Does it sell advertising? Is it sponsored by a drug company? Could there be a conflict of interest?

• Is the information based on scientific evidence, with medical facts and figures referenced to published research studies in reputable journals, with advice/opinions set apart from information based on research results?

• Is any information provided about the risks or side-effects associated with the proposed treatment?

• Is the site regularly updated? It is important that medical information is current, with the most recent update clearly posted.

Finally, Professor Ernst urges all web-seekers to ask themselves whether the treatment in question claims to 'cure' cancer. 'A lot of very valid treatments, like acupuncture, work alongside conventional treatments, and their value in alleviating symptoms and side-effects such as nausea and pain, especially in late-stage disease, is supported by stronger and stronger evidence. I would be much warier of treatments claiming to cure cancer, considering them to be crossing the line between the responsible and irresponsible, and I would automatically distrust anyone who suggested I should stop what I was doing medically and follow their therapy.'

He also recommends extreme caution if all 'evidence' of effectiveness is based on a single study or research paper. 'Look instead at the totality of the evidence for and against. Are positive findings supported by different institutions and authors, or is all the research emanating from the same place?'

171

Professor Ernst's last word on the matter? 'If it sounds too good to be true, it probably is!'

## 55. *Know when to express reservations, and when to keep them to yourself and offer 110 per cent support...*

In *Grace and Grit*, the American psychologist Ken Wilber details the five-year cancer journey he and his wife embarked upon after she was diagnosed with breast cancer. It was a journey not only in a metaphorical/psychological sense, but in a literal one: they travelled to Europe for the most radical form of chemotherapy available anywhere in the world, tried meditation, yoga, vegan diets, and later travelled to New York and embarked on the controversial Gonzales/Kelley programme of pancreatic enzymes swallowed down with dozens of different supplements.

Ken Wilber's conclusion as to whether you should voice any concerns you may have about a particular cancer plan that a friend or loved one is set upon, orthodox or unorthodox, boils down to one thing: timing. 'If you are genuinely sceptical about a particular treatment,' he advises, 'voice that scepticism during the period that the person is trying to decide whether or not to do the treatment. That's being honest and helpful. But if the person decides to do the treatment, then shelve your scepticism and get behind them 100 per cent. At that point your scepticism is cruel and unfair and undermining… They don't need to hear about the dangers of the radiation or chemotherapy or Mexican clinic they've chosen, a choice usually made with great difficulty after long deliberation.'

*I'm very supportive of people choosing to do whatever they want to do. We know so little about cancer, I'm of the view that when anyone feels they have had enough of the conventional way, that it has exhausted all it has to offer them, and says 'to hell with that', we should support them all we can, whatever they propose doing. Even if it's nothing at all, and simply allowing nature to take its course.*
Rabbi Julia Neuberger

## *… while encouraging them to check out what they intend doing with their medical team*

It's important to recognise that 'natural' remedies can have side-effects, as with any regular drug (shark's cartilage, for example, can cause nausea and vomiting, while megadoses of vitamin C can provoke diarrhoea), or they may work against other medicines. There is concern, for example, that some herbal remedies, such as St John's Wort, may interfere with chemotherapy by activating liver enzymes which may break down the toxins faster. And a new research study from Yale School of Medicine in Connecticut suggests that black cohosh, frequently taken to alleviate menopausal problems, could compromise the effects of radiotherapy.

According to Dr Sosie Kossab, 'even vitamins and antioxidants could have a detrimental effect on chemotherapy regimes. We just don't know. It's possible, for example, that antioxidants may compromise effectiveness by protecting cancer cells more than normal cells. One antioxidant vitamin has even been linked with more, not less, cancer, so vitamins aren't the unalloyed force for good that many people assume they are.' It's telling, for example, that doctors at the Memorial Sloan-Kettering Cancer Center in New York specifically advise against taking vitamin supplements during chemotherapy (with the exception, in some cases, of folic acid), as they fear that their antioxidant action might interfere with the process of cancer cell death.

Since dramatic weight loss can be a feature of some cancers, doctors may also express reservations about cancer diets which outlaw so many foods (no fat, no sugar, no salt, no dairy, no alcohol, no acid-forming foods) that they are almost invariably very low in calories and protein.

# When the going gets tough

After battling through all the treatments, news of a recurrence can hit harder than the initial diagnosis, especially if many years have passed in which friends and family, as well as the individual, have reached an accommodation with the cancer, a state of seeming equilibrium. And then, the news from hell: It's back, and in one of the no-hope sites that take a person in one single heart-lurching leap to the far end of the cancer-care continuum where doctors stop talking about percentage chances of cure and start talking instead about 'management' and 'quality of life' and 'putting you in touch with your palliative care team'. It's very hard and very scary: the fear, the shock, the sense of all that treatment undergone for so little return. When cancer comes back, faith, hope and trust can take a real battering.

*My sister Alice had been living with breast cancer for 14 years, and though we only knew for the last nine, we had become comfortable with what was going on, had lapsed into this false sense of security because she had been clear of any symptoms for so long. Then my sister Victoria phoned us when we were on a Christmas holiday abroad and told us that the cancer had spread to her lungs and her brain. The news came from a clear blue sky and it knocked us all sideways. It was a huge shock, a huge adjustment, particularly for her. For a while, she was so devastated she was beyond reach and none of us could comfort her.* Lord Falconer of Thoroton, the Lord Chancellor

*Strange things knock you for six, such as arranging your child's birthday party and wondering if it will be the last. Wondering if your fragile bones will be strong enough to withstand the bounce of*

176

*a landing hot-air balloon, a long-held dream. Wondering if, when the time comes, you will have the capacity to handle your death, and the pain of your family in witnessing it. Hating it each time someone you have met with cancer dies, and that throat-catching feeling that you could be next.* Sally Hamilton

## 56. *Seek out the small pleasures*

'All that matters is not to lose the joy of living in the fear of dying,' wrote Maggie Keswick Jencks, the inspirational founder of the Maggie's Centres, a wonderful resource for people with cancer, now springing up all over the country. 'Life can get desperately sad and terribly serious,' agrees Maggie Bisset, my palliative care nurse. 'It's easy for people to lose sight of the person they used to be, the things they enjoyed.'

Dame Cicely Saunders, inspirational founder of the Hospice movement, has always insisted that paying attention to the small pleasures is a central part of compassionate nursing care. On one famous incident, she was conducting a ward round with a group of doctors when she stopped a nurse and asked her to be sure to remember that the patient in the bed in the corner would like to have her toenails painted. In something of the same spirit, you, too, can help friends find space for a little frivolity in their lives: a good gossip, an afternoon home movie, a small manageable shopping spree (if only on the internet), a cup of hot chocolate in a favourite café with lavish dollops of cream on top.

*You have to be very careful you don't start living your illness – doing nothing but living, breathing, talking cancer. Caron, through her quest to find a complementary way of living alongside her orthodox treatment, discovered the art of living in 'the now' – for that very moment. She made a point of doing something every day purely for enjoyment. She'd go out for lunch, or to an art class, or have a feel-good therapy session or go out to the cinema with a friend. She lived for seven years after her diagnosis and it wasn't all angst, all struggle; there were lots of happy moments, lots of laughter, and much love amidst it all.* Gloria Hunniford

*When my sister, Ruth, knew that she had terminal breast cancer, she said to me that she wanted to enjoy the little things in life, as well as the big stuff. So I took her clothes shopping whenever she wanted (she developed a passion for bias-cut Ghost dresses), and also to get her eyebrows shaped, and we ate large quantities of cake together. Her favourite flowers were sweet-peas and lavender, so I always tried to bring her bunches of both, and if she felt the urge to discuss George Clooney or red lipstick or the contents of Vogue (which was quite often), then that was what we'd sit and chat about. But when she did want to talk about the savagery of what lay ahead – of dying, when her twins were still babies, when she had so much to live for – then I did not try to change the subject. And I'm so glad that nothing was left unsaid.* Justine Picardie

*We have a friend with a cancer that has now travelled to her bones and every week four of us women play tennis together. We have a hysterical time. She serves underarm, and because she now plays so gently, she actually wins a lot of points, as the rest of us are stand-ing too far back. It's clearly causing her some pain, but she says it gives her a normality; when she's playing tennis, she's not thinking about anything else. Just living in the moment and enjoying the camaraderie of friends, she says, has made the game a beacon in her week.* Mary-Ann Wilmot

# 57. *Respect the decision to decline further treatment*

When it's clear that the cancer is now incurable, and any ther-apies on offer will henceforward be palliative – that is, designed to relieve symptoms and make the patient comfortable – many people check out from further treatment. While the right to decline treatment will be respected without question by their medical teams, families may find such a decision much more difficult to accept, even to the point of putting much intended or unintended emotional pressure on the sick person to change their mind. Friends can often do a great deal at this point to act as go-betweens and to support the interests of patients, who may not feel strong enough to resist and make the case for themselves.

*The time I have spent with young people as patron of the Teenage Cancer Trust, and the experience of being with my mother and mother-in-law and a close friend, has taught me that this illness affects people in very different ways. I have learned not to be judgemental, to accept that everyone's needs differ – teenagers, for example, who see the world in a very different way from us adults, may need to be explosively angry or to completely withdraw. After my mother was diagnosed with very advanced cancer and refused all treatment, I realised that if I was going to be any help at all, I would have to let go of my fear, and my assumptions. With cancer, there can be this pressure to fight it right to the bitter end, but a time came when my mother didn't want to fight it any more and when we who were closest to her needed to let go of that wish ourselves in order to let her know that what she wanted was absolutely OK.* Duncan Goodhew*

*A close friend (33 years old, devastatingly handsome with no surviving family) has just been diagnosed with a grade IV glioblastoma deep within his brain and has decided not to even embark on treatment. Coming to terms with this decision has been extraordinarily difficult. We all like to think we would have the fight deep within us, at whatever cost to our dignity and remaining weeks or months of life, but after a week of soul-searching, and listening to both my friend and my far more rational husband (whose mother died of cancer), I reached the inevitable philosophical conclusion that it was not my right as a friend and colleague to force his fight;*

*moreover, if the fight did not come from deep within him, and him alone, then it would never be won. I have had to recognise that I am not the one with the worst kind of brain tumour in my head and to respect his decision that, knowing he has, at best, less than a 1 per cent chance of survival, he wants to live every last moment he has to the fullest.*

*Today Hendrik has nothing except an occasional headache. He does not want to start the denouement now, or to think that his last few weeks of freedom and dignity will be robbed by hospitals, operations, chemotherapy and drugs in a fruitless effort to prolong his life. He consulted experts, he informed himself. And however hard it has been to accept that Hendrik has turned his back on his only hope of survival, it has made me realise that courage is also knowing when, and what, to fight.*

*It is his wish that his legacy to the world will be an MRI machine – a fight his friends will win on his behalf.* Zoe Appleyard-Ley

*I know from my work as a chaplain that families can feel very threatened, very upset, if the patient is not seen to be doing everything within their power to stay alive. They take it very personally. They don't understand that the prospect of having to endure another round of side-effects from treatment, which the patient knows about far better than a relative can ever do, makes them want to call a halt. In such a situation, I would advise relatives and close friends to support anyone who chooses to stay alive in the best pos-*

*sible circumstances rather than for the longest possible time.* Rabbi Julia Neuberger

## 58. *Record a video or tape while your friend is still strong enough to participate*

After someone dies, especially a close friend, sibling, partner, child or parent, it can be desperately distressing to find you can no longer recall their voice or their laugh, or the way they looked. Any recording may be too painful to be enjoyed soon after the event, but it can be tremendously comforting in the years that follow.

*We made a video for my friend's children of her doing all those mundane everyday things – washing up, gardening, ironing, story-telling – to help the children remember what their mother did on a day-to-day basis, and what she looked like. We also had her speaking to camera with family members and old friends about her childhood, schooldays, first boyfriends, first meeting with their father, etc. It only took a few days to complete, but it gave them precious images to remember her by when she was healthy and 'normal'-looking rather than ill and exhausted and wasted, as she became at the end, and gave enormous solace after she died.* Mary Shearer

*After her dad died, one young person told me that the thing she wanted most that she could never now have was the memory of the sound of his voice. She felt guilty that she couldn't recall such a vital and unique part of him and she hadn't been able to find him on any of her relatives' video films, as he was often the one behind the camera and, not being naturally given to issuing directions or making comments, remained both an invisible and an inaudible presence. Wouldn't it be wonderful, we agreed, to hear the laughter of someone you want to remember.* Frances Bentley

*My mother died when I was very small. But despite the fact that I didn't know her at all, I've missed her all my life. Not only when I was little, but now, when I'm breaking new ground, different ground, doing new things that she never had the chance to do. I often wonder how it would be if I'd known her just a little, inconsequential things like what made her laugh and what her dreams were for the long term she never had. When she died, she and my father were building a house, and I would love to know what she would have put in her unplanted garden. If my mother had had the time and the technology to do that, I know I wouldn't miss her half as much as I do.* Joanna Cary

# 59. *Offer to help prepare a memory box*

There are some wonderful boxes you can buy, and beautiful

tissue paper and ribbon with which to fill and decorate them. While for some people this is a very private project, others find it a companionable undertaking, with lots of light-hearted moments and laughter, as well as poignant reminiscences. You can seek out the boxes together and discuss what you might put in them, with you helping to hunt out small mementoes and keepsakes.

**Ideas of things to put in memory boxes**

• Favourite colour swatches.

• Postcards of paintings or places.

• Photographs, including the disastrous ones.

• A lock of hair, the imprint of a lipstick kiss.

• A handwritten list of the happiest days of one's life.

• Things that tell a child about a time before they were born, when the parent was a child, or a teenager or before they were married.

• 'Personal treasures': things that were precious as a child and have been kept.

• Books enjoyed as a child with little notes slipped in to mark favourite passages.

• Favourite sweets as a child (Barrett's sherbet fountains, sugar mice, gobstoppers, pear-drops, Parma violets, favourite-coloured Smarties or Liquorice All Sorts).

• Letters and pictures that the children have written.

• Memories of what the children did, said or wanted packed in their lunch boxes; letters to Father Christmas; lists of their favourite friends, toys, books and songs; the sort of things a grandparent might tell a grandchild about his or her parents.

• Items of jewellery, gloves, belts, etc.

• Lists of hopes and dreams.

• Packets of seeds to plant.

• Recipes of favourite dishes.

• Theatre/opera/circus/football match programmes.

• A desert island disc of favourite music selections, along with the associations they conjure/reasons for choosing them.

• Tapes of the person reading much-loved passages of poetry or prose; and of meaningful sounds from the bark of a dog to the rustle of silk taffeta 'because that's my enduring memory of my mum as she leant over to kiss me goodnight in bed when she was on her way out to a party'.

• Favourite scents and evocative smells such as patchouli or lavender or a Gitane cigarette that conjure a part of the past.

• A signature lipstick or nail varnish.

**Find further ideas plus boxes, etc, from the charity Winston's Wish at www.winstonswish.org.uk**

*Memory books and boxes can become family treasures. So can plans for memorial services, or an anniversary celebration. When people you love die, it can be a tremendous comfort to know that you are remembering them exactly as they would have wanted. Friends and family can offer ideas and the guarantee that wishes will be carried out in the years to come.* Esther Rantzen

# 60. *Have those difficult conversations*

Is death the 'final failure' to be fought every step of the way, or the last stage in an individual's cancer journey? It's clear from the people I talked to in connection with this book that some accept that their lives are coming to an end and are able to be very open about it, sharing their fears and hopes, and making calm and careful preparations for the future of those left behind. Others find it hard to grasp that the latest developments mean they will not now be cured, and prefer not to think about death at all (perhaps out of the superstitious belief that to dwell on it might in some way hasten the event), instead concentrating all their attention on the present and putting their remaining energies into living and getting well – holding out hope right until they die. 'We never had that straightening-out conversation, because my husband was fighting it every step of the way till the day before he died,' said one woman regretfully. 'We had both convinced ourselves that he was getting better, that he would pull through.'

While it can be stressful for relatives and friends when someone who is dying starts talking about getting better and making plans for the future, people working in palliative care say it can be equally stressful for a dying person to be surrounded by people who are relentlessly cheerful and strenuously avoid the one subject that is staring them all in the face.

In her inspirational and compassionate book *Intimate Death*, one of France's best-known palliative care experts, Marie de Hennezel, writes: 'The dying person knows. All that's needed is some help in being able to articulate that knowledge. Why should it be so hard to say? Isn't it because everyone else's distress makes it hard to talk, and so the dying person has to protect them? Our experience confirms that the person who can say to someone else "I am going to die" does not become the victim of death but, rather, the protagonist in his or her own dying. It is a moment of standing up straight again, and of the return of an inner strength that nobody else knew was there. The person who can say "I am going to die" can conduct that departure, organise it…'

Friends who are unafraid can be marvellously supportive at this point, both in facilitating a dying person's wishes and in acting as a safe sounding board for whatever they want to say. If relatives are inadvertently making it harder for the dying person to talk about what they are facing, to look back at their life and to make plans for tying up loose ends in the time they have left, and you are uncomfortable broaching the subject yourself, try tactfully suggesting that the family might arrange for your friend to see a counsellor or chaplain, or to talk to a Macmillan nurse.

*When a good friend of mind was dying of leukaemia, we talked about it. Death. This big thing that we all have to do, that most of us don't normally cater for in any shape or form. 'How does it feel to be dying?' I asked him. I didn't feel coy talking about it. He said it was clearly not the thing he wanted or planned, he was leaving his wife and children, it was a nuisance, and he'd rather not be going, thank you very much, but it didn't feel like a disaster. It was a major disaster for his wife and children and friends, of course. But he had this complete acceptance. He said he was aware of a curious completeness. He wrote a letter the day before he died which was read out at his funeral, saying there was something in every situation to be relished, something life-enhancing, even in the shadow of death. That was his conclusion.* Monty Don

*I wanted to help John address the natural fear of dying, during which it became clear that what he really worried about was the effect on his wife Lindsay, their daughter Ellie and his unborn child, Hope. He said if there was one thing he asked of me, it was to make sure I did what I could to look after them, and make sure Ellie never forgot him and that Hope got to know him a little through his friends. Ellie used to make me tell funny stories about him, and read to her the stories he used to read to her. She talked about the silly drawings he did for her and the looning around. She didn't forget him for a single day. She just didn't have enough days to live since, tragically, she died a few years later of the same non-hereditary illness.* Alastair Campbell

# 61. *Help with forward planning…*

Explicit end-of-life conversations with professionals, family and friends when a person knows that their time is limited can come as a huge relief, leaving them free to enjoy the time that is left without crowding anxieties and morbid preoccupations. Areas that may require attention and/or action might include:

• Arranging a power of attorney, along with a separate bank account to allow the surviving partner to withdraw money (all assets are frozen at death).

• Finalising the will and getting it signed (see the CancerBACUP guide to making a will and leaving a lifeline).

• Considering guardianship of the children, remembering to ask their nominated guardians whether they consent to the arrangement.

*When my best friend knew that her cancer was terminal, she became obsessed by the future of her two young children. She was very anxious that her husband would re-marry and have more children, and that they would be cheated out of their inheritance. She felt that she had been more or less solely responsible for setting the family in its good financial stead as she had managed all the finances, mortgages and, indeed, even her husband's own finances, and she feared that if he were to dissipate their combined wealth, her own children would be the poorer. She wanted me and her other great friend to try and make sure, as trustees of her will, that this did not happen. Sadly she died without signing her will, so it has been almost impossible to fulfil this function on their behalf.*

*As for injunctions to 'look after' the children when she was gone, she was in such a dither about her time of departure that by the time it was apparent she really was about to die, she was rather incoherent. We hope that by acting in loco parentis – by continuing the tradition of family dinners on Sundays, and including them in various bucket-and-spade-type seaside holidays – we are keeping to the spirit of her wishes, but it would have been 100 per cent easier for all of us if those wishes had been enshrined in writing. And I now wish that I'd been more proactive.* Alison Andrews

## ... including life and end-of-life decisions

• Help your friend to have conversations with professionals and family members about what they want. Do they want to die at home, in a hospice or in a hospital? Who do they want with them? What sort of service would they like? Burial or cremation? Find ideas and inspiration in material produced by the Natural Death Centre (call 0871 288 2098 or visit www.naturaldeath.org.uk), a charitable organisation that aims to help improve the quality of death by supporting those dying at home, and their carers, and by helping people arrange inexpensive, family-organised, environmentally friendly funerals.

• Who might they like to see? They may choose to see people

191

they have not seen for years, to say important things that have remained unsaid and to make preparations – practical, emotional and spiritual – to die. A good close friend can do much to facilitate this, from tracking down friends they may have lost touch with years ago to finding sources of spiritual succour.

• Get in touch with community nursing care services (through a GP or palliative care nurse) so your friend can get to know those nurses who will be coming into the house as and when the need arises to provide help with washing, pain relief and symptom control; a couple of familiar names and faces can be very reassuring.

• If control is important, your friend may welcome the opportunity to make a living will or advance directive – see *A Guide to Living Wills*, which can be downloaded free from the Patients Association website (www.patients-association.com). This is best done in the presence of a key medical practitioner who can anticipate what might be experienced in the circumstances and can specifically cover for those eventualities, always bearing in mind that a person is free to change their mind at any point.

• Even if the intention is to stay at home to the end, circumstances and wishes can change. People often seek the relative privacy of a hospital or hospice room as the house fills up with visitors, so why not offer to accompany them on a visit to your local hospice or hospices? You can check out hospices for end-of-life care just as you can check out schools for your children or antenatal facilities. In a big city, there may be a choice of two or three. It can be comforting to know the option is there, and that the place is already in some way both chosen and familiar.

In addition to the many NHS hospices on which your health professional can advise you, there are also ten Marie Curie hospices in the UK, providing the best possible care to people with cancer at no cost to patients or their families. Each offers specialist care for in-patients and outpatients, along with daycare and home visits. To find out about hospice services in your area, phone Hospice Information (0870 903 3903), which publishes a directory of hospices and palliative care services; Marie Curie has a useful website (www.mariecurie.org.uk) giving links to its ten hospices.

*I'd always ask people who know that they may die soon what it is they desperately need to do. And whole-heartedly encourage them to do it. It may be something as simple as feeling the rain on their face or their bare feet on the grass. Or it may be more complicated and plainly medically inadvisable – like going to India, as was the case with one dear friend of mine. We talked it over for some time and I urged her to go.* Rabbi Julia Neuberger

## 62. Keep the patient central to decisions concerning their care and their affairs and the life of the family

Sometimes with the best of intentions, people try to 'spare' the dying person involvement in troublesome family issues, such as money problems or an adolescent crisis, when often it hurts more to be sidelined and to feel one no longer has any part to play in the life of the family.

Preserve a sense of normality. Try not to jump in and take over those myriad day-to-day tasks they would normally do themselves. If you can, always ask your friend directly whether something you propose might be helpful, rather than filtering the request through others and leaving your friend out of the discussion. Offering what you can when you can, and accepting a 'No' with good grace, may help your friend to feel that they are still capable and effective and in control of their life. Let them tell you when they need assistance.

*The important thing to remember when someone you love is living with cancer or is terminally ill is to help them live the rest of their lives. However ill they are, do whatever you can to help them to feel in control of their daily life, to have dignity, and whenever possible to laugh together.* Sir Elton John

Finally, it is isolating enough being ill without having nursing staff and doctors talking about one's care to relatives in separate rooms; when people are whispering behind closed doors, it's easy to imagine the worst. People who had acted as carers towards the end of life told me they had found it was nearly always better, and much less frightening, to openly involve the dying person in discussions about their care.

## 63. *Know your place in the scheme of things*

Palliative care nurse Maggie Bisset observes that there is often a natural process of withdrawal and closing off as the final stages of any illness set in. 'To begin with a person might lose interest in going out and want to stay at home, then they may lose interest in going outside and will want to remain indoors, and so on, until finally they retire to one room and even just to a bed, and eventually retreat into themselves as they prepare to let go.'

As horizons close, and strength diminishes, the number of visitors who are truly welcome tends to dwindle to a few trusted presences. Some people cannot bear others to see them so ill and changed, to see the shock in the eyes of friends who last saw them when they were relatively well. Or it may be that they only feel comfortable with one or two people who are instinctively attuned to their needs, and nobody else will do.

'Unfortunately,' says Maggie Bisset, 'this may be a time when they are inundated with calls and visits. When a person is dying, people often want to be with them all the time, and cannot bear the thought of leaving them alone for a second. When everyone is queuing up for a last goodbye, this can be so exhausting for the patient that when all the farewells have been said, they often rally and have a second wind.'

The actress Patricia Hodge advises asking yourself a few honest questions about whether you merit a place at the bedside, or would be more use sending gifts and/or supporting the primary care-givers.

*My experience has shown me that when your health starts to fail, your horizons shrink and just staying alive becomes the most monumental effort. That's the time to be honest about your place in that person's life and react appropriately. When an old friend recently became very sick, I recognised that, although our friendship went back a long way, I did not deserve a place at her side, so I sent flowers and cards instead.* Patricia Hodge

*So what can friends do? The answer is fairly obvious. Know when the sick person wants you there, and know when they don't. Ask them what they want. If it's nothing, or if it's privacy, respect that. Think about the family, worry about them, but know when to*

*leave them alone, too. Their suffering is always greater than yours, and needs the greatest support.* Alastair Campbell

## *Useful gifts*

• A CD player with a remote control so it is not necessary to get out of bed to change discs or turn the volume down.

• A meditation/relaxation tape that you can listen to together, and that can be played whenever your friend feels anxious, tense or sleepless. The Bristol Cancer Help Centre's online shop (www.canhelpnow.com) has a wide selection, and also sells sleep-enhancer sprays and aromatherapy candles.

• A home visit from a hairdresser, an aromatherapist, a healer or reiki practitioner for a gentle hands-on treatment that gives another form of contact beyond the clinical.

• Club together with friends to buy the entire collection of a comedy series (such as *Ab Fab*, *Six Feet Under*, *The Vicar of Dibley*, *Blackadder*) or drama (*The West Wing*), historical costume dramas (Dickens/Jane Austen, etc) or serious documentaries to while away the hours and hours.

*Time dragged quite desperately. A lot of people sent brilliant videos.*

*Best of all was the person who gave us Simon Schama's History of Britain. It helped to have a bit of a theme. Not to mention 26 episodes. He watched every single one of them. I also bought him a tape of the Iliad, which he loved and listened to at least five times.* Sarah Poland

• A visitors' book for hospital/hospice visitors.

*When my cousin was in hospital and very sick, and was dying, lots of family were coming to visit from abroad. Since only two of us were able to be at the bedside at any one time, it was hard to keep track of who had come to visit and who still needed to be contacted. I bought a visitors' book and kept it by the bed so that visitors could write what day and time they had come and leave little messages or sketches or even polaroid photographs. It stopped the family worrying about who had or had not heard, and who had or had not visited, and the entries became a great talking point that took some of the pressure off making conversation.* Annette Elizabeth

Palliative care nurse Maggie Bisset also recommends a baby alarm, so that the sick person can make their needs known without having to shout or get out of bed, and everyone else can get on with their lives, together with:

• An electric fan, to help alleviate feelings of claustrophobia and fluctuating temperature.

• A baby toothbrush, to keep the mouth moist and clean.

• A book for writing down dreams, which can be very vivid in the last months and weeks of life.

• Spare pillows and sheets ('people never have enough').

## 64. *As horizons shrink, bring the world into the house or the bedroom…*

Bring the outside inside by introducing nature into the house: place a few beautiful stones or shells or branches along window sills; pot up early narcissus and hyacinth bulbs; and fill vases with buds in spring, tall strong sunflowers (and bunches of aromatic herbs, especially mint) in summer, beech leaves in autumn.

Help arrange a change of scene in the bedroom, whether by moving the bed or chair to afford a different view out of the window, or simply by arriving with freshly laundered sheets (and making up the bed), a talking book or an amusing anecdote, or by making a meal tray attractive with fresh flowers.

When reading becomes an effort or concentration is hard, it's a real pleasure to be read to. Offer your services in this way and always discuss what your friend would like to hear first. And perhaps set up a regular hour when you drop by each day – or again, set up a rota – so you can get through a book reasonably swiftly. Also investigate talking books and talking book libraries.

*Towards the end, Jack didn't want to go out much. People would come and cook us meals and I reinstated the Friday-night tradi-tional Shabbat dinner, gathering a collection of old friends and family and people we hardly knew. Jack loved his house, loved the ritual of lighting the candles, loved to see everyone eating, loved to hear laughter and conversation. One Friday, I invited the American director and the choreographer of Thoroughly Modern Millie, whom he hadn't met before, to join us; another time a young Israeli journalist; and on one occasion a Nepalese asylum-seeker; and it made for a rich mix. They brought a new colour.*
Maureen Lipman

## *… and turn hospital or hospice rooms into more homely environments*

Bring photographs, a home duvet and pillows, candles, cushions, throws, sarongs or stretches of fabric, a favourite mug or cup and saucer, beautiful glasses, appetising home-cooked food.

# 65. *Include the children*

With the house full of concerned well-meaning adults, it is easy for the children to get excluded. Friends clustering and chatting around the bed can create a physical barrier. So hold back when the children get home from school. Some children find it difficult to initiate contact, and may need to be given errands and small chores that give them a reason to be in the room.

• Move a computer or television and video player into the bedroom so children can watch a programme with their parent.

• Give a child a task, such as mashing up a banana, filling a hot water bottle, making tea, spooning juice or soup, massaging hands or feet, or painting a mother's nails ('toes were better,' comments one friend, 'as they were far enough away for my rather particular friend not to be able to see how badly they were done!').

• Instigate a game of cards or chess, or have a giant jigsaw on the go on a table by the bed.

*We brought the computer into Simon's bedroom so that the children, who had tended to stay away, were always in and out, tapping away, without having to sit around the bed, feeling awkward and making conversation. Simon wanted them close by, to have that sense of life going on all around him, rather than continuing somewhere else without him.* Sarah Poland

*I was sad when I found out that my mum was ill. But then I found out there were lots of things we could still do together – like have cuddles and read stories and watch TV together, and I can kiss her on the forehead.* Freddie Stebbings (aged 9)

## 66. *Care for the carers*

When cancer happens, it happens to the whole family. Stepping in and supporting the primary care team by offering simple services, such as sewing name-tapes on to the new school uniform, mowing the grass, sourcing and wrapping Christmas presents, can be hugely supportive to those whose attention and energies must now be otherwise engaged. Don't just turn up and, worse, require feeding. Visits should impose no obligations. Offer to make the tea yourself. Bring supper or cakes for the family.

Because of the fear of alienating those around them, it is often the few people closest to those nearing the end of their lives who take the brunt of their fear and anger and bitterness and despair. This can be very emotionally wearing. Principal carers are under an unimaginable degree of strain, often for weeks and months at a time, and their emotions can easily be magnified by exhaustion, worry and fear. Offering yourself as a willing pair of hands before patience runs out and reaches breaking point is a gift indeed.

Vicky Wells, co-founder of the Cancer Support Community in San Francisco – who has had cancer herself and has also been a carer, and thus has the advantage of both perspectives – has eloquently summed up the especial strains and pressures on the shoulders of these unpaid, under-appreciated and un-applauded attendants.

*I've been in both worlds – I've had cancer and I've been a support person. And I would have to say that it is so much harder being a support person. Because, at least for me, when I was dealing with my own cancer, there were a lot of moments of sheer beauty and clarity and grace and reordering of priorities in life, and a re-appreciation of the beauty of life. And I think that, as a support person, that's really hard to find. The cancer person has no choice but to stay with it, but the support person has to choose to hang in there all the time. And it was real hard for me, as a support person, to get over the sadness, or get over the feeling of walking on eggshells around the person, or living with their treatment choices… it's like an emotional roller coaster.* Vicky Wells, quoted in *Grace and Grit*

*Some days, I felt so confined it was like I was under house arrest. I didn't have the energy to organise my own expeditions, but I was so grateful to friends who took me out: who came and collected me, bought me lunch, took me swimming or to an art exhibition. They'd ring me and say, 'We're coming to collect you', or they'd fix it a few days in advance in order to give me a chance to arrange cover. That would give me something to hang on to, something to look forward to.* Sarah Poland

*Partners need lots of support – particularly to be angry and rail against the unfairness of the world, and to be dragged off to the pub to have 'a nice time', at least superficially.* Moira Smyth

• Offer to stay overnight at home or at the hospital, or to keep the sick person company for a stretch of time, taking on instructions for nursing care, so the carer can have a reasonable amount of time off and, as important, get a good night's sleep.

• Offer to stay with your friend while the carer goes out and has a massage that you have pre-arranged, or a swim or beauty treatment, or goes to a movie.

• Explore respite options such as Crossroads Care. This is a voluntary organisation that aims to support carers. Care attendants are trained in basic nursing and can meet the needs of an ill or disabled person for a period of time so that the carer can have a break. There are Crossroads Care attendant schemes in many areas. Discuss your needs with the area organiser, if you think you may need this help. The number is in your local phone book, or phone head office (0845 450 0350).

Marie Curie nurses can also provide care for patients in their own homes, day or night, allowing patients to remain at home when they might otherwise have to go into a hospital or hospice, and giving the regular carer the chance to have a break or sleep. Get information about this service, which is free, through community/district nurses or your GP, or by contacting Marie Curie Cancer Care (020 7599 7777).

• Find out about relaxation classes on the carer's behalf. Many cancer support groups run relaxation sessions, or GPs may offer classes at their surgeries. Counselling can also often help dissipate pressure-cooker feelings: get help from the Cancer Counselling Trust (020 7704 1137), Carers UK (0808 808 7777), or an organisation called 2Higher Ground (01684 850456; www.2higherground.org.uk), which supplies coaching to carers, or former carers, of cancer patients, 'to help them regain clarity and control, discover new outlooks and choices, reassess priorities and feel better able to cope with the present and whatever the future may hold'.

• Drive the carer to the hospital, particularly if it is quite some way and they do not have transport, or are having to do the drive on a daily basis. People with advanced cancer often end up in hospitals far from home, and their biggest pleasure is seeing their families, who may only be able to get there infrequently.

• Offer to take the children off for treats and, even better, sleepovers.

• Organise a rota of close, trusted friends to be briefed together by the carer/district nurse so they can take over for a few hours every day, and stay some nights.

*When an old friend of mine was in the final stages of her illness, she developed terrible bedsores. The people from the social services were so unreliable that she cancelled them and said that her greatest luxury was having her neighbour call in three times a day to help her husband turn her over in bed.* Clare Murray

## 67. *Take good care of yourself*

It's a truism that you must take care of yourself first and foremost if you are going to be able to take care of anyone else. Yet people at the sharp end typically ignore their own needs. Overwhelmed by the all-consuming neediness of the person they are nursing, and very often the large numbers of people coming into the house or the hospital, many come dangerously close to burnout. If this is you, explore respite care options (or ask the very next person who asks what they can do for your partner/parent/friend/child to explore them for you) and put yourself first for a change.

*I forgot to look after myself. For months, my schedule was crazy. I would visit one parent in one hospital and one parent in another hospital and work all day and then fit in two more visits before doing live TV in the evening. I never went to the gym, never sat down to eat a proper meal. It may feel incredibly selfish to be thinking about yourself, and your needs, when someone very close to you is desperately ill, but you have to maintain your health and strength, to keep yourself together and going.* Gaby Roslin

*I would do it again unhesitatingly under the same circumstances. But I would do it differently, with more of a support system in place, and with a clearer understanding of the devastating toll that being a full-time support person can take.* Ken Wilber, *Grace and Grit*

> **NB** As you find yourself taking on more of a nursing role, ask your district/community nurses for instruction about how to move and handle bed-bound patients so as not to cause any damage to your back.

# 68. *Be sensitive to spiritual needs*

If the dying person expresses a need for spiritual comfort or companionship, Richard Chartres, the Bishop of London, suggests finding a non-lethal member of whatever faith is appropriate who is licensed to talk about God. I asked him what he meant by 'non-lethal' and he replied: 'Someone who is secure enough not to impose their own spiritual agenda, who is not over-talkative, who is overflowing with non-oppressive confidence in his or her own faith and can respond sensitively and appropriately to the questions that may be asked of them.' Such a person might best be found by ringing your local hospice as, through long experience, the hospice movement tends to attract and employ people who can offer real succour and solace to the dying, and who are genuinely unfrightened of what lies ahead for all of us.

In addition, the Bishop advises friends and family who genuinely want to help to be sure they are not exploiting the moment to foist their own spiritual agenda. While I had marvellously supportive and sensitive help from my brother Matthew, who is a lay preacher, and from Kit Chalcraft, a retired vicar friend of the family who sent amusing notes and snippets from books and inspirational passages from a whole range of surprising sources, I also had to fend off some very well-meant advances by those presumably hoping to win celestial brownie points – including the suggestion of a last-minute conversion to Roman Catholicism.

*There's no room for fantasy and fairy tales and easy glib assurances. Or even for facts. You can't tell people things that they don't, in some part of their being, already know. If you are genuinely* *trying to help, the first thing you have to do is come to terms with your own mortality, your own fear. Then give the person space in which to ask their questions. Don't impose your own. One of my friends who always took the Dorothy Parker strategy of 'Tell it to me slant' would say things like 'Shall I need another mackintosh?', which might mean 'How long have I got?', so I'd invite another question and we'd slowly edge towards a more explicit question that I felt better qualified to answer.* Richard Chartres, Bishop of London*

*Spiritual care is not about imposing one's will, or one's views, on someone. It is about listening. It is sometimes about dealing with the hard questions. It is sometimes about honesty, truth so sharp that it is painful. But it is never about saying, 'I want to pray with you', or any other imposition of self.* Rabbi Julia Neuberger

Richard Chartres makes the point that there is often an unexpected reversal of the give-and-take dynamic that generally prevails as people approach the end of their lives. Having for so long been accustomed to being the helpers and providers and people on the giving end, we may be surprised to discover that the dying person is in a position to do a good deal more for us than we could ever do for them.

*However frail, a dying person is much more than a dwindling presence in a bed. People who are dying have great power and*

209

*authority, can do huge good and are often in a better position to help others than they have ever been. It's a very creative time. Part of the work of dying is to liberate people – people who are terrified or constipated or embarrassed or paralysed by survivor's guilt – from their fears. People who are dying can pass on very precious gifts to their own children that no one else can possibly do.* Richard Chartres, Bishop of London

## 69. *Even the very ill can sometimes be tempted by delicious food and drinks or even illicit treats*

Chocolate, champagne, asparagus, Belgian chocolate milkshakes that can be sucked through a straw, small cubes of pineapple kept in the fridge, fresh fruit sorbets made into ice cubes…

Even in the final stages of the disease, there can be small foodie pleasures. When my friend Liddy was near the end of her life in the Wellington Hospital, it was June and very hot, and her mouth was so dry and uncomfortable that a mutual friend slipped out and bought her a strawberry Calippo, which she polished off with such relish she upended it to get the last of the juice.

AT THE SAME TIME, BE CAREFUL NOT TO MAKE FOOD DEMANDS. Because it is one of the very few things people can still do to help a very ill person, the preparation and eating of food can become disproportionately important. Community care nurses tell how conflicts and tensions can quickly flare up around food, and how a loss of appetite becomes threatening even though it is quite normal in the final stages of any illness. Friends and relatives need to understand this and not take the rejection of what they bring to the bedside, so lovingly and thoughtfully prepared, as a rejection of them.

*Someone has lent me their silver ice-crusher. It looks like a 1920s cupboard and makes a sound like a concrete mixer. Drinks have become piles of glistening pink, yellow and orange icy water.* Julia Darling 'in person', Blog, 28 March 2005

*When my friend was rendered virtually paralysed by his cancer in the last few days of his life, the one thing he really missed was his nightly joint. One evening, he asked me to close the door to his hospital room, take out his 'special tin' from his backpack, roll him a joint and blow the smoke into his mouth. As a marijuana virgin and non-smoker, this proved to be a farcical and frustrating experience for both of us, as I fumbled and farted around trying to complete my task with speed and any sort of aplomb. It ended with ME high, but both of us in fits of giggles, and eventually both of us wet our pants. Excellent.* Dawn French

211

## 70. *Keep talking, keep touching. Even when talking back is not possible, the senses of touch, smell and hearing remain acute right to the last*

Bring in freshly mown grass or new hay, a single fragrant rose, even the family pet (animals are welcome in many hospices).

*When someone is very ill, people stop touching and holding them. Partners in particular may pat them or stroke them, rather like a pet, but the physical aspect of their relationship, the intimacy, goes. However, it doesn't have to. There can still be a place for more sensual touching and contact right to the end of life.* Maggie Bisset, palliative care nurse

*When my younger brother James was dying of mesothelioma in the intensive care ward of a New York hospital last year, he was on a ventilator attached to tubes and monitors, and we could only communicate by touch. So I'd sit there for hours at a time squeezing his hand and he'd squeeze back. He was a doctor, a brilliant intellectual, cerebral man, but at the end what he found most comforting, was simply to be touched and held. I spent a lot of time, sitting with him, talking to him, about his family and his children, of whom he was so proud, about how much he'd achieved, about how he was surrounded by all the people who loved him. I bought some lavender oil as an antidote to all the clinical hospital smells, that I knew he would find evocative of summer holidays, and I massaged his feet. I kept his mouth moist with a sponge dipped in minty water. I put lip balm on his lips. When you are gravely ill and supremely uncomfortable, these tiny things are disproportionately nice. I did it for both of us. For him first and foremost, but also for myself. I needed to feel I had done everything I could have possibly done, to have a sense of completeness.* Tessa Jowell

*Caroline would say, 'I am not battling with cancer, I am living with cancer.' She wanted to carry on as normal, enjoying her home and her garden and her four children and her ten grandchildren, and was very determined to remain in control right up to the very end. We were all round the bed when the nurse whispered to me, 'You might like to tell her she can go.' So I did, and a few moments later she stopped breathing. I was very moved, and everyone there was impressed. It was an inspirational death. It is the one certainty on this earth, that we are all going to die, and it was a gift to those of us who loved her to have witnessed such a quiet and, yes, easy death.* Tony Benn

# Survivorship

After the shock arising from the diagnosis and, very often, the outright trauma of treatment, there can be a real moment of elation in realising that, yes, we have pulled through, turned a corner and come out the other side – if not exactly fighting fit and well, and with none of the old easy assurance of an indefinitely long life ahead, then certainly armed with a much more positive sense of a future to look forward to.

*It is now nearly four weeks since the amazing news that the scans showed no cancer in me. The feelings of relief, delight and gratitude were enormous, and I think Tiff and I cried every day for a week. Those feelings continue to return like a wave at random times, with varying levels of emotional impact: sometimes I just grin, and sometimes I can barely hold it together. Sometimes I am delighted just to be sitting on my own, well and enjoying a rugby match or a beer; at other times I want to publish my story, take all the doctors to the Ritz and sell my house in aid of cancer research.*
James Ewins

As with all clichés, the current cancer favourite – 'cancer is a word not a sentence' – has an element of truth. Increasingly people are surviving their cancer, living with it, in the way that people with diabetes or epilepsy live with their conditions. Given the pace at which medical research is proceeding – not a month goes by without news of some radically new drug transforming survival hopes for someone – certain experts predict that by the year 2015, cancer will have become yet another survivable disease, a chronic condition that we will die with rather than from.

However long we've got – still the great unguessable, whatever the doctors say – we embark, post-treatment, on a new stretch of our lives that the Americans have taken to calling 'survivorship'. It's a term that has yet to catch on in Britain, where we are rather more superstitious about standing up and declaring ourselves cured. It seems a preposterous enough presumption to be booking a holiday, buying new summer clothes, taking out a year's subscription to a magazine or renewing a football season ticket without crowing about having beaten a disease that, as one person put it, 'always seems to get you in the end'; writing books with bullish titles like *No Time to Die*, as my old boss and ex-editor Liz Tilberis (1948-1999) did, seems just a tad too triumphal, inviting fate to knock us sideways yet again.

While we may not choose the 'S-word' in relation to ourselves, the concept of survivorship is a useful one in that it implies that this is an acquired skill requiring practice rather than simply a passage of time the other side of treatment. For most of us, learning to live with cancer, rather than somehow existing despite of it, is a huge adjustment. We come out of the long dark treatment tunnel into a period of what the cancer doctors call 'watchful waiting', marked by increasingly infrequent clinic appointments, and scans and tests at longer and longer intervals. And in place of the light, joy and general jubilation we were led to expect, we often find yet more anxiety, yet more fear, yet more uncertainty. Even with the best prognosis in the world, surgery for cancer can never be as straightforward as having our tonsils out, although everybody around us may let out a deep sigh of relief, and unhelpfully assume that it's OK now, they can all go home; everyone and everything can return to normal.

*After my surgery my mum and my mother-in-law said, 'So it's all gone now? It's all better now?' They thought that if I'd had it cut out, that was the end of it. So I'd say, 'No mum. It's not like that. It doesn't just go. I've got to learn to live with it.'* Nazira Visram

*People who don't have cancer themselves want to hear you say that you're cured. They don't want to hear you talk in the same careful and measured way your doctors talk, that there's no sign of it now and the tests are clear but, of course, with cancer one can never be sure, one can only hope. No, they want to hear it's all over and done with, that you're fine and they can go on about their lives and not worry about you; no ogres are lurking behind bushes or around corners.* Treya Killam Wilber, *Grace and Grit*

*I was ten years old when I broke my arm playing football and they found a tumour on the bone. It really wasn't a big deal. Children accept everything as normal. I'm the youngest of five, and suddenly I was getting plenty of attention. Every time I went to the hospital we'd go and have lunch and ice cream. Then I had my operation and I can remember that, afterwards, I felt stronger-tempered. My sister had breast cancer – mastectomy, chemotherapy and all the horrors. Recently she had the all-clear. 'How "clear" do you feel?' I asked her. 'How clear is "all"?' 'Well,' she said, 'I've been taken off the books because today it's clear, and last year, and the three years before that, but I never stop thinking maybe they've got it wrong.'* Monty Don

217

After the high drama of the diagnosis and the exigencies of treatment, being sent away for a period of watchful waiting can be the most nerve-racking part of the ordeal. As the accumulated tiredness, tension and terror take their toll, people who weathered their treatment brilliantly, rising to the challenge of losing their hair and whatever else was thrown at them, can fall apart quite spectacularly.

*About a year after I finished treatment, I got deeply depressed. Sort of 'What the fuck's the point of living?' My wife found it the last straw. 'After everyone has done so much for you…' she'd say. She was so utterly unsympathetic that I found the aftermath even more isolating than my cancer had been. And the professionals weren't much help, either.*

*My hospital was brilliant on surgery, brilliant on chemotherapy, but 100 per cent useless on aftercare. Nobody told me that this might happen. Nobody warned me. Yet now I learn that it's very common. And in a way it was harder to cope with than the chemo.*
Charlie Wilson

Many people I talked to spoke of feeling 'very wobbly' in the months after their treatment ended and they were discharged from hospital care. 'It's definitely not a yippee moment,' said one. 'You can suddenly feel abandoned. You're still not feeling 100 per cent well, but everyone expects you to be up and on your feet again.'

218

*I am now feeling a lot better, starting to get fit again, the mental fog is lifting and I just hope it is for a long while. But it doesn't take much to make me shaky.* Suzanne Long

Although the sense of urgency and emergency fades, many people talked of being left with a bone-deep fatigue that persisted for months, even years, and a host of barely articulated anxieties, together with mood changes that took them completely by surprise. No one, they said, had warned them that they might be left feeling scarred, maimed or disfigured physically or emotionally by the experience; or that it was perfectly usual to suffer fear, anxiety, flashbacks, even panic attacks. As one person put it, 'Weeks and months were punctuated by fits of crying and depression, with some really good days scattered in between.' It can take years, not months, and certainly not weeks, for the memories and high anxiety to fade and for cancer to begin to become a background presence in one's life. It's an ongoing process during which friends can either continue to be a huge support or unwittingly make assumptions that can make things a whole lot worse.

# 71. *Step right in. Your support may be most vital now*

If, as is often the case, the principal supporters are themselves exhausted post-treatment and need their own recovery time, and compassion fatigue has set in elsewhere, offers of help may now be more gratefully received, and more useful, than at any time before. Several people commented that it was when they were no longer under the close supervision of their medical team that they felt at their most vulnerable and alone with their cancer, and most in need of emotional and practical support – even though they often felt they had relied on their friends enough and should now be able to manage. Being discharged from active treatment signalled their re-entry into the real world, and made them feel they no longer had any right to impose their needs on anyone.

*While out walking, I bumped into a friend who was cooking me supper in the evenings and I felt like such a fraud. If I was well enough to be walking down the road enjoying the sunshine, I was well enough to take back the reins of my life in other ways. I felt I should be doing more for myself, that I shouldn't still be needing that level of help. After all, I had completed my treatment so the worst was over, but the truth was I still needed support, more than ever in fact.* Nazira Visram

*Life goes on as normal for 99 per cent of your friends, of course it does, but this increases your sense of isolation from your old life. And while there can be no going back to your old life (can there ever?), there is a yearning to go back, as this seems safer than the future.* Sally Hamilton

Making the transition from cancer patient to person living with cancer means adjusting to a new, rather different kind of future: much as we would like to, we cannot, as so many assume, just go back to normal, because normal itself has changed. And while a new normality will establish itself over time, and can be every bit as good, it must be, by definition, different: one that accommodates uncertainty, the unsettling reality that, even after treatment, and with the most cutting-edge technology available, doctors will never be able to offer a 100 per cent guarantee that every last trace of the cancer has gone.

*What I need now is a doctor who will tell me that he's run my body through an electronic mincer and can tell me without any doubt that there are this many cancer cells remaining, that they will be killed off on precisely this day, that there are no rogue cancer sites in my toes or my ears or my kidneys and that Blue Boy will win the 4.30 at Kempton Park.* John Diamond, *C: because cowards get cancer too*

*I had the 12th chemotherapy session yesterday, 26.2 miles completed in marathon terms. But the exhilaration of crossing the finish line is not quite all it could be due to the inherent uncertainty of treating and curing cancer. In fact, emotionally, it has been quite a difficult milestone, with the doctors taking care to stress that even though my bone marrow results came back clear, it does not guarantee there is no lymphoma anywhere in the bone marrow.* James Ewins

*The way I look at it, it's a bit like being a trout on a fish farm. Every year, some sod is going to hook you out, make you go back to hospital, submit you to blood tests. Come December time, I still get anxious, worry it's going to be bad news. They know in the office. They say 'He's going to London', and leave it at that. And I finished my treatment 26 years ago.* David Moar

*Fear is the big enemy we have to deal with. That and living with a degree of uncertainty. I used to find it very difficult. Now I look at my future as an elastic thing. I concentrate on the present.* Dee Dee Hope

> **NB** Cancer treatments such as radiotherapy and chemo-therapy can be followed by months of draining fatigue; see CancerBACUP's booklet *Coping With Fatigue*.

# 72. *Plan normalising activities which underline that a friend with cancer is much more than just a 'cancer patient'*

Lots of people I spoke to said they suffered something of an identity crisis after they had been signed off by their specialists: for so long their cancer had become the central talking point, the focus of all their common efforts and energies, that they were left feeling unsure about who they were when it was all over and they were discharged back into the real world. This disorientation was all the more pronounced if they had either given up or taken an extended break from work. So much of our identity is wrapped up in what we do, rather than who we are, that when illness forces a prolonged or permanent break from a job, we suffer losses that go beyond income. Instead of the lawyers, teachers, nurses, students, builders or bricklayers we once were, we are reduced in the world's eyes to 'the person with cancer' – a label that, by extension, may also be attached to other members of the family, with equally unwanted effects. My youngest daughter, for example, started a new school in the September before my cancer was diagnosed. She was still very much the new girl, still feeling her way, had yet to forge firm friendships and was longing for nothing more than to be one of the crowd, when suddenly, and much against her will, she was singled out for special treatment and became 'the girl with the mother with cancer'.

Friends can do much to help reinforce and/or bring out other aspects of the person – encouraging him or her to discover a new energy or creativity by taking up a musical instrument, joining a choir, orchestra or local drama group, signing up for art classes, photography workshops, yoga holidays or creative writing courses such as those run by the Arvon Foundation (www.arvonfoundation.org). Children who have had cancer might be encouraged to join the Brownies or Scouts, or take up a new interest such as pottery or street dancing. Whether you are a child or an adult, being in a group composed entirely of new faces, where no one has any assumptions about anyone else, can be remarkably liberating. Friends can also act as vital go-betweens with work colleagues and further-flung friends who may need encouragement to get back in touch; by making the first overture, they can also help put a stop to the inevitable round of rumours and Chinese whispers that can make a person's re-entry into the everyday world, and especially the workplace, much more difficult than it needs to be.

*I went to a wedding the other day and someone I knew vaguely, not very well, came up and said, 'I must introduce you to this woman who had cancer ten years ago.' I knew that it was well meant, and that it was supposed to be encouraging for me to meet a long-term survivor, but I felt uncomfortable, so I said, 'Look, I'm sure she's very brave and thank you for the thought, but no.' That's happened to me four times now. I feel like I've got this big label round my neck screaming 'Cancer victim', when all I want is for people to treat me normally, as no one and nothing special.* Anna Blackman

*Everyone asked me whether I was going to go off and join a hippy commune, or go to Morocco. They were expecting this changed new person to emerge. But the only thing I wanted to do was to recover my old life. 'Normal' is such a downbeat word, but that's what I*

*wanted more than anything, what I absolutely craved: to go back to normal, to find normal again.* Charlie Wilson

*Work was very therapeutic for both of us in the ten years Georgie had cancer. Because we found it best to keep busy, she was always very keen to get back to school; it became a sort of sanctuary where she didn't have to think about her illness, where her friends accepted her without questions and she could be herself.* Nicola Horlick

# 73. *Don't be surprised if your friend, and friendship, undergoes radical change*

After the great pioneer of humanistic and transpersonal psychology Abraham Maslow suffered a near-fatal heart attack in 1968, he lived for two more years, referring to the stretch of blissful and purposeful calm that followed as his 'posthumous life' – shot through as it was with a bittersweet sense of his own mortality, and marked by an absolute determination to use the time left to him to the full.

'Priorities change. They line up differently,' observed Ruby Wax after spending several mornings with breast cancer patients at the Royal Marsden Hospital. And it's true: as their health and strength return, many people speak of having a new clarity about what really matters in their lives, of time being too finite and too precious to get bogged down in unimportant details. At the same time as re-evaluating priorities and friendships, they often feel impatient with, and discard, all that seems trivial. I myself often talk about BC (before the cancer) and AD (after the diagnosis) because it did indeed seem that at that definitive moment at four o'clock on Friday 26th November 2004, someone had come along with a big black pencil and drawn an indelible line under my old life, changing everything utterly.

*We are all so busy. After the cancer, some of my busy-ness fell away. I stopped rushing through my life. I found the time to stop and stare, to really focus on those things that nurtured my soul.* Heidi Locher

*You develop a core of steel, an impenetrable core, a toughness, which allows you to deal with everything, but it's not necessarily a good thing. It makes me much more ruthlessly committed to whatever I'm doing, a workaholic.* Sam Taylor-Wood

*If, as a child, you had cancer and you survived, it stays in your system. Even now, nearly 40 years on, I still live for the day; everything is a stumble from moment to moment. I'm very bad at planning for the future, to the extent that there can be some catastrophic results. I'm very, very irresponsible in that way. The present is just all that there is. There is just the moment. You can't count on anything else.* Monty Don

If it is too much of a presumption to suggest, as some self-appointed amateur psychologists do, that people should look upon their cancer as 'a gift' or 'the best thing that ever happened to them' ('Cancer is NOT the best thing that ever happened to me,' wrote Sally Hamilton furiously, 'I cope with it; it demands great reserves of courage and fortitude that seem to run dry every now and then, it has NOT yet been a spiritually enriching experience, although I must admit I have read books and been to workshops that might not otherwise have occurred to me'), when people do talk of their cancer being the best thing that ever happened to them – which is their prerogative, not anyone else's – what they are usually expressing is gratitude for being jolted out of stagnation and complacency, and having their lives infused with a new sense of purpose and direction.

*It shook me up in a right old way, my cancer did. I am convinced that, without it, I would still be leading the same joyless existence in the same dead-end job with the same unsatisfactory relationships, just waiting for retirement and for the whole damn thing to come to an end.* Kenny Potter

The same transformative changes may happen to those who accompany close friends or family members through what has come to be called their 'cancer journey', however it ends.

*I'm definitely a different person as a result of Georgie's illness. Less*

*selfish and materialistic. I do considerably more for charity, for other people, than I would have done if Georgie had not had leukaemia. I recognise that the reason I had her for ten years more than I might have done is down to all those people who worked so long and so tirelessly for leukaemia research, both in the laboratory and raising money.*

*It doesn't have to be leukaemia. Anything Georgie might have wanted me to do, then I'll do it. I'm vice-president of the UK Committee for Unicef, for example, because she was so upset during the Sudan crisis when children were dying for lack of food, to the point that she saw her own bone-marrow transplant as a waste of money that could have been better spent on life-saving meals for those children.* Nicola Horlick

*It was all about Georgie. It was always about Georgie. She was my older sister and was diagnosed with leukaemia at the age of two, soon after I was born. So for the first ten years of my life, all the family's attention was on her, especially when she relapsed, which happened twice. Then she'd be in hospital for a long, long time. Our nanny wasn't big on treats or taking us out. So my treat would be if Georgie came home or I went to see her in hospital.*

*After Georgie died, I found it fairly lonely, to be honest. I bottled everything up. As you grow up, you get closer and closer to your friends – they can help you take your mind off it, to escape. But at that age, my friends couldn't help. Later I had counselling, which really helped. I'd sit and cry for hours. And now? I'm a much*

228

*more open person. It's bizarre. But it feels right, it feels good.*
Alice Horlick (aged 16)

## 74. *As energy returns, help the transition from patient to survivor by finding a positive focus*

There are many ways of using one's experiences of cancer – particularly the negative ones – in a positive way, especially now that, after centuries of invisibility, patients are suddenly becoming a sought-after commodity. Our opinions are canvassed and our views are listened to, and patient representatives have become key presences on hospital committees and steering groups. 'If I jumped up and down in an effort to get anything changed,' said one member of my medical team, a touch ruefully, 'it wouldn't be nearly as effective.'

In this new era of patient power, any of us can use our experiences of healthcare (good and bad) to help improve the provision of services both locally and across the UK – whether by taking on the local hospital authorities about the cost and availability of parking, or campaigning to reduce waiting times for chemo and radiotherapy treatment. Actively engaging with politicians and decision-makers to effect change that will benefit others can be very empowering.

Talk to your friend to see if they might like to use their experiences in this way. If they are interested in joining an expert patient programme or user group, contact Pals (the patient advice and liaison service) in your local hospital, your local Cancer Network office (look in the telephone directory) or join the Macmillan CancerVOICES network, which is helping to shape the future of cancer care across the country.

Other ways in which people have been able to put their experience to good use, so enabling them to feel more like a survivor than a victim, include raising much-needed awareness in their local communities. Nazira Visram, for example, who had always shrunk from putting herself forward in public, was encouraged by her husband to stand up and be counted and so help to counteract the negative image of cancer that prevails in many Muslim communities.

*In the community I come from, we don't talk about illness and we don't talk about cancer. Cancer equals death. It's shameful. It can affect your social standing, your children's future. People suffer in silence. Even the extended family may not know. There were times when I felt like a freak; when, even if people weren't avoiding me, I felt that they were.*

*So now I'm feeling stronger, I've decided that, instead of pretending it hasn't happened, I'll try and help them understand a little more, open doors of communication. These days I'll go and talk, do what I can to raise awareness. There's so much fear. As it's the elders within the family who have the dominant role, I like to address the subject through them as a way of seeking support and approval. I'll stand up and talk to the seniors at their clubs and say 'I have had cancer and I was unlucky, but I am still around', and I give them the opportunity to ask as many questions as they need with the view that the information will filter down and become more acceptable.* Nazira Visram

Just being open about their cancer, and offering support and guidance to people going through the nightmare of diagnosis and treatment themselves, can be as important for the person on the giving as the receiving end.

*As a survivor of bladder cancer, with a one-in-four chance of making it past the first few months, I realise I am living in a very exclusive club. Seven years on, people seek me out as somebody who their recently diagnosed friends with horrible prognoses can talk to, as a sort of living example of survival against the odds. I had marvellous treatment, the best, and if I can put something back, I'm happy to do it. I'm not squeamish. But the rest of the world is.* Charlie Wilson

*My entire life changed in the short space of ten minutes, when I was told both that I had colon cancer and that I would have to have a non-reversible colostomy. All I could remember was my own mother saying, 'I would rather die than have THAT operation.'*

231

*Although the stoma nurses were wonderful, what would have helped hugely at the time would have been the chance to talk to someone who had had the operation, who could have told me that it wasn't the end of the world and given me advance notice of the nitty-gritty details that I had to pick up as I went along. Twelve years on, I now offer myself as a befriending presence to people facing the same operation through my local hospital and GP's surgery. It feels good to be using my experiences to help those going through the same ordeal.* Rhodanthe Selous

Or you may like to join forces with others to set up your own support group through the auspices of Cancerlink (now a part of Macmillan Cancer Relief), which provides training and back-up for people starting groups, supplies good practice guidelines and organises annual conferences in Manchester and Scotland. Your presence in these groups as a 'supportive other' will encourage other carers to come, and can be a shining light to those in similar situations.

Or your friend may be provoked by some experience of their own to start something that (with your help and enthusiasm and support) snowballs and snowballs and snowballs…

*Big C was conceived one cold, wet afternoon looking out of the window of Ward 8 South at Charing Cross Hospital. I was a gypsy, with my clothes in my suitcase, constantly travelling to the hospital and back to my family in Norfolk or my wife's family in Kent to*

*recuperate for a few days before the next chemo. My life was controlled by doctors and consultants, blood tests, X-rays and CT scans. Having survived the treatments, and being a mere six-stone weakling, I was determined to make sure that in the future people in Norfolk would not have to travel 120 miles for their treatments, but could have access to the very best care locally.*

*In September 1980, I got together with a friend and the Big C – a name we borrowed from John Wayne – was born as a charity. In 25 years, we have raised over £8 million, funded cancer wards, specialist nurses, countless bits of equipment for diagnosis and treatment, research programmes and even our own Chair of Cancer Research at the University of East Anglia. It's been great fun, but also a lot of hard work. However, when we see the bricks and mortar, or articles published in the medical journals as a result of research we have sponsored, it makes it all worthwhile.*
David Moar

Putting one's energies, and even grief, into a project or greater cause can also be helpful for quite another kind of survivor.

*I found strange comfort in making up silly verses in my head when I couldn't sleep or woke up in the night or was driving the long distances to the hospital to see Jack. Weird really, but I wrote 30-odd animal poems and then never wrote another. Now I'm putting them together with illustrations by friends in a book to*

233

*raise money for a myeloma charity. A sample:*

> *The lemur cub was crying.*
> *'Why so sad?' I ask her,*
> *'I'm a homesick lemur with a broken femur,*
> *And my mum's in Madagascar.'*

Maureen Lipman

*I try to keep the memory of John and his daughter Ellie alive by working with Leukaemia Research, running and cycling and swimming and speaking to generate money and awareness. I don't know if it helps or not. People tell me it does, and I like to think they're right. But when I'm doing it, I feel he's there, still doing what he always wanted to do as a journalist, which was to try to make a difference.* Alastair Campbell

*After our daughter, Anna, died, Megs, my wife, and I set up the Willow Foundation for young adults, aged from 16 to 40, with a life-threatening illness. The idea was to have 'Anna's Special Days'; opportunities to escape the pressures of their daily routine by realising a lifelong dream or regaining some precious normality. In six years, the charity has grown to 15 full-time members of staff and 90 volunteers. We have sponsored 800 of these special days so far, and it's become incredibly important, not just for these young adults, whose needs have traditionally been rather overlooked, but for both of us as well. It keeps us in contact with Anna in a very vital way.* Bob Wilson

# 75. *Be thankful for the good that comes out of a crisis*

Through everything – the good, the bad, the ugly and the unrelievedly awful – is the enduring bond of real friendship, forged in crisis and tested by often extreme circumstances. What's for sure is that whether the friend you have supported goes on to enjoy several more years or even decades of life and outlives everyone, or dies from their disease as so many still will, the experience will have left you in countless small but important ways the richer for it.

*It was a very long-running thing. Ten years after all. People had their own lives to lead. They'd appear in a real crisis, send flowers and presents and come and visit. But Georgie's best friend's family were unbelievable. They could have backed off from the friendship. We would have understood. If Georgie didn't survive, and we all knew from the beginning that she could die, it was going to be very traumatic for their own daughter. But they were there right up to the last day of her life. They were there when we turned off her life support machine. They changed her and got her ready and put on her nightie. They were incredibly supportive, very kind. And the links continue. We have just celebrated Georgie's friend's 18th birthday. Having been through all of that together, there is an unbreakable bond between us.* Nicola Horlick

*A friend of mine threw a dinner party for me once I'd come through my second lot of chemotherapy, and invited my 12 best friends, and it was such a generous thing to do, and quite emotional, because seeing them all together I realised how much they had done not just to make my life bearable through the bad times, but to transform the bad into something good, at times even better than it had been before. And I went to a shop called Party Time in Camden Town and bought them all little Oscar statuettes and we had a little ceremony and speeches, and I presented them all with Oscars for Best Supporting Friends.* Anna Blackman

## ... and what it teaches us

What's quite clear from the dozens of people I spoke to who had all at some point stepped into the breach is that when you take on the role of befriending someone with cancer, whether related to you or not, whether initially a very close friend or not, the learning never stops.

*It's being a secure presence, that's what I learnt from my sister. I was so frightened. I was the younger sister. She was the older sister/ mother figure. I took her to the Bristol Cancer Help Centre and drove her to hospital appointments. I had the potential to be helpful, but I couldn't bear to hear what was really on her mind. When she'd say things like 'I don't know what to do about the children', the blind panic would descend. There was so much fear, I wasn't able to deal with it in the way I would now. Eighteen years on, I've become much better in hospital and treatment situations. I used to be quite frightened of the medical professionals. Now I'm not. I'll spend hours researching things for friends, taking the doctors on, asking questions on their behalf.* Felicity Kendal

However well or distantly we know someone, when we hear they have been diagnosed with this most dreaded of all diseases, if we choose to roll up our sleeves and do whatever we can to lighten the load on their shoulders, we will take something of enduring value away with us, whatever the eventual outcome.

Befriending a person in need is a skill. Even the Macmillan and specialist cancer nurses say they never stop learning, that they get better at it over time, adapting their approach in the light of what they learn from each new patient. Hardly surprising, then, that we, too, are continually learning as we go along; that the lessons we learn from being with one person, whom we may at times feel we have failed, we can apply with the next. And with one in three of us destined to join the ever-lengthening cancer statistics, what's quite certain is that there will always be someone else out there who needs our support, someone else to help…

# About Macmillan Cancer Relief

**Macmillan Cancer Relief**
Registered charity number 261017
89 Albert Embankment, London SE1 7UQ
www.macmillan.org.uk
Tel 020 7840 7840
CancerLine 0808 808 2020 / email cancerline@macmillan.org.uk
Textphone for deaf and hard of hearing people 0808 808 0121
For general enquiries, or to be put in touch with your regional
office, call Macmillan on 020 7840 7840

Macmillan Cancer Relief is delighted to be involved with *What Can I Do to Help?* which so honestly and clearly explains how people can be supportive of friends who are coping with cancer.

People often find themselves at a loss to know how to help – whether through fear, embarrassment or lack of understanding. Worries about doing 'the wrong thing' can sadly mean sometimes friends do nothing at all. However, through her experiences, and those of others, Deborah has shown just how much a friend can do – from simple, practical favours, through to deep, on-going emotional support. Relationships can become stronger, and more meaningful. Friends can make a real difference.

Macmillan Cancer Relief helps people with cancer in many ways, and can help you if you are supporting a friend too. We provide expert care and emotional support, offering a range of innovative cancer services and are at the heart of improving cancer care throughout the UK. You may know Macmillan best for our nurses, but we provide a wide range of services.

**Macmillan nurses** provide expert care in hospital and at home, keeping abreast of new treatments and are concerned with feelings as well as physical health. They use their specialist skills to provide emotional support, pain relief, symptom control, information and advice to people living with cancer from diagnosis onwards. They don't just help the person with cancer, but are there to support the family and carers too.

**Macmillan specialist consultants and doctors** deliver cancer treatment and care, undertake research, and advise and teach other health professionals.

**Other Macmillan health and social care professionals** work across a range of disciplines, many delivering cancer treatment to patients (e.g. radiotherapy) or improving quality of life following treatment (e.g. occupational therapy). Our social workers help people who need social, practical and emotional support. All these professionals have expert knowledge to help people affected by cancer.

**Macmillan cancer care centres** are healing environments for people at all stages of their illness. Designed and created by

Macmillan specialists, they use architectural and design principles which have been shown to improve people's response to treatment and help them get better, faster. Over 100 projects have now been completed, including new-build schemes, conversions and extensions, both for NHS Trusts and for independent hospices.

**Macmillan information and support services** When you, or the person you're caring for, are upset or frightened, it can be hard to take in information – or remember to ask the doctor the questions you want answers to – perhaps about treatments, or caring for someone at home. Macmillan can help, either directly with quality-checked, up-to-date information about all aspects of cancer, or by suggesting someone else who can.

Our **Macmillan CancerLine** provides free information and emotional support for people affected by cancer – the people with cancer themselves, their families, and their friends. We provide information about living with cancer, caring for yourself, or someone you love, and also where else to turn to find further sources of information or guidance. You can reach the service via telephone (freephone 0808 808 2020, Monday to Friday, 9am to 6pm), via a textphone service for deaf and hard of hearing people (0808 808 0121), by email (cancerline@macmillan.org.uk), or by writing to CancerLine, Macmillan Cancer Relief, 89 Albert Embankment, London SE1 7UQ. A link to the Language Line interpreting service allows us to speak to callers in 150 languages. If you need to leave a message out of hours, we will call you back.

We also fund and start up **information and support centres** – mainly based in hospitals but also such places as libraries and GP practices. These often offer face-to-face support, as well as information and someone to guide you through it all. Macmillan CancerLine and our website can tell you if there is a centre near you.

**Local support groups** There are hundreds of self-help and support groups around the UK run on a voluntary basis by people who have experience of cancer, either directly or through a family member or friend. Groups offer a range of emotional and practical support and some offer complementary therapies. Some are supported by Macmillan (we provide resources and training), but we can also put you in touch with many more. Just call the CancerLine to find out about groups near you.

We also offer **financial help and advice** to people struggling with the additional costs associated with having cancer, such as hospital parking, or fares to and from treatment. Some people face extra heating and clothing bills. If working, having cancer, or caring for someone, may also mean a break from work and a significant loss of income. Macmillan can help.

People with cancer can apply to Macmillan for a small **grant** to help meet specific costs associated with having cancer – for example, for a short break or a washing machine. You (or the person you're caring for) will need to ask a health or social care professional, such as your Macmillan nurse or social worker, to complete an application on your behalf. Please call Macmillan CancerLine for further details on our eligibility criteria and how to apply.

The **Macmillan Benefits Helpline** is a telephone advice service for people with cancer, their family and carers who need help to access benefits and other kinds of financial support. Calls to the helpline are answered by experienced benefits advisers who can check exactly which benefits and other kinds of financial help people are entitled to claim and help fill in necessary forms. It's open 10am-5pm Monday to Friday, except Wednesdays when it is open 12-5pm. The number is 0808 801 0304.

We also have a very useful booklet, *Help with the Cost of Cancer*, which tells you more about benefits, grants and financial help generally. You can request it (free) through the CancerLine or the Benefits Helpline.

Practical and emotional support for carers is provided by a growing number of **Macmillan carers schemes**. If you are caring for someone living with cancer at home, you may find there are times when you need some support yourself. Or you

242

may simply want an understanding listener, such as a Macmillan CancerLine adviser. You may need advice or information. Or you may need practical help, such as someone trained in caring for people at the end of their lives, who will care for your relative or friend so you can have a break. Macmillan CancerLine will find out what is available for you in your area.

**Macmillan education, development and support services** help Macmillan professionals and other health and social care professionals develop their skills – and deliver cancer care to the very highest standards. There are now seven Macmillan education units within universities, Macmillan lectureships, financial awards for continuing education, a professional resources programme and two practice-focused research units.

Macmillan supports **CancerVOICES**, a network of people affected by cancer who are helping shape the future of cancer care across the UK. Macmillan also supports people who have experienced cancer services to get involved in planning and improving services through the NHS Cancer Networks.

**Help us to help others…**
… by volunteering, taking part in an event or giving a donation. To find out more, please contact Macmillan on 020 7840 7840, write to us, or visit www.macmillan.org.uk/supportus
Thank you.

# Cancer charities, support groups, information sources

### 2Higher Ground
*Puts carers of cancer patients in touch with coaches who will help them to cope with uncertainty, to balance competing priorities and to gain a clearer outlook.*
**Tel** 01684 850456  **Fax** 0700 580 3158
**Website** www.2higherground.org.uk

### ACT (Association for Children with Life-threatening or Terminal Conditions and their Families)
*Provides information on support services for families and produces various publications, including a charter setting out the facilities that should be available.*
**Address** Orchard House, Orchard Lane, Bristol BS1 5DT
**Information line** 0117 922 1556  **Fax** 0117 930 4707
**Email** info@act.org.uk  **Website** www.act.org.uk

### Beating Bowel Cancer
*A national charity working to improve bowel cancer awareness among the medical profession and the general public. Provides information about the disease, its symptoms, what to do if diagnosed and what treatment choices are available.*
**Address** 39 Crown Road, St Margaret's, Twickenham, Middlesex TW1 3EJ
**Tel** 020 8892 5256  **Nurse advisory line** 020 8892 1331
(Tues, 9.30am-5pm; Fri, 9am-1pm)  **Fax** 020 8892 1008
**Email** info@beatingbowelcancer.org  **Website** www.beatingbowelcancer.org

### Brain Tumour Foundation
*Support network, plus education and information resource for patients, their families and healthcare professionals.*
**Address** PO Box 123, Tewkesbury, GL20 7YT
**Tel/fax** 01684 290439  **Email** btf.uk@virgin.net

### Breast Cancer Care
*Dedicated to providing support and information to women with breast cancer as well as to their families, partners and friends.*

**Address** Kiln House, 210 New Kings Road, London SW6 4NZ
**Helpline** 0808 800 6000
**Email** info@breastcancercare.org.uk **Website** www.breastcancercare.org.uk

## Bristol Cancer Help Centre
*Offers a residential therapy programme for people with cancer and their support-*
*ers which is complementary to medical treatment. The programme includes relax-*
*ation, visualisation, meditation, counselling, healing, art and music therapy,*
*bodywork and nutritional advice.*
**Address** Grove House, Cornwallis Grove, Clifton, Bristol BS8 4PG
**National helpline** 0845 123 2310 **Fax** 0117 923 9184
**Email** info@bristolcancerhelp.org **Website** www.bristolcancerhelp.org

## British Colostomy Association
*An information and advisory service. Emotional support is given by helpers with*
*long experience of living with a colostomy. Free leaflets and local contacts available.*
**Address** 15 Station Road, Reading, Berkshire RG1 1LG
**Tel** 0118 939 1537 **Helpline** 0800 328 4257
**Fax** 0118 956 9095
**Email** sue@bcass.org.uk **Website** www.bcass.org.uk

## CancerBACUP
*Helps people affected by cancer, their families and friends. Qualified cancer*
*nurses provide information, emotional support and advice by telephone or letter.*
*Provides booklets, factsheets, a newsletter, website and CD-rom.*
**Address** 3 Bath Place, Rivington Street, London EC2A 3JR
**Freephone helpline** 0808 800 1234 **Fax** 020 7696 9002
**Email** info@cancerbacup.org **Website** www.cancerbacup.org.uk
**Scotland office** 0141 553 1553

## Cancer Black Care
*Offers practical and emotional support, addressing the needs of black and ethnic*
*minority people affected by cancer. Telephone or drop-in service available. Provides*
*one-to-one counselling and advice on grants, benefits and general welfare.*
**Address** 79 Acton Lane, London NW10 8UT
**Tel** 020 8961 4151 **Fax** 020 8961 4152
**Email** info@cancerblackcare.org **Website** www.cancerblackcare.org

## Cancer Counselling Trust

*Provides in-person and telephone counselling for cancer patients, their families, friends and care-givers.*
**Address** 1 Noel Road, London N1 8HQ
**Tel** 020 7704 1137  **Fax** 020 7704 8620
**Email** support@cctrust.org.uk  **Website** www.cctrust.org.uk

## Carers UK

*Campaigns for a better deal for carers, informing them of their rights and what help is available; trains and advises professionals who work with carers.*
**Address** 20-25 Glasshouse Yard, London EC1A 4JT
**CarersLine** 0808 808 7777 (Weds and Thurs, 10am-12pm and 2pm-4pm)
**Tel** 0207 490 8818  **Fax** 0207 490 8824
**Email** info@carersuk.org  **Website** www.carersuk.org

## CLIC Sargent

*The UK's leading children's cancer charity. Provides advice, information and support, as well as practical help and financial assistance, to children with cancer and their families. Services include healthcare professionals, cancer centres and grants.*
**Address** Griffin House, 161 Hammersmith Road, London W6 8SG
(Also offices in Bristol, Edinburgh, Glasgow and Belfast)
**Tel** 0845 301 0031  **Website** www.clicsargent.org.uk

## Colon Cancer Concern

*Concerned solely with colorectal cancer. Aims to sustain the normal quality of life, increase the cure rate and to prolong survival by campaigning for screening and treatments of proven benefit.*
**Address** 9 Rickett Street, London SW6 1RU
**Tel** 020 7381 9711  **Infoline** 0870 850 6050  **Fax** 020 7381 5752
**E-mail** info@coloncancer.org.uk  **Website** www.coloncancer.org.uk

## Crossroads – Caring for Carers

*More than 200 schemes across England and Wales which provide a range of services for carers, including care in the home (by paid, trained care workers) to enable carers to have a break.*
**Address** 10 Regent Place, Rugby Warwickshire CV21 2PN
**Tel** 0845 450 0350  **Fax** 01788 565 498

**Website** www.crossroads.org.uk **Scotland office** 0141 226 3793

## Cruse Bereavement Care

*Offers help to people who have been bereaved, in any way, whatever their age, nationality or belief. Free counselling service. Opportunities for contact with others through bereavement support groups and advice. Nearly 200 local branches.*
**Address** 126 Sheen Road, Richmond TW9 1UR
**Helpline** 0870 167 1677 **Fax** 020 8940 7638
**Email** info@crusebereavementcare.org.uk
**Website** www.crusebereavementcare.org.uk

## Foundation for Integrated Health

*Promotes research into and development of integrated healthcare. Also supports the complementary healthcare professions to develop national standards of training.*
**Address** 12 Chillingworth Road, London N7 8QJ
**Tel** 020 7619 6140 **Fax** 020 7700 8434
**Email** info@fihealth.org.uk **Website** www.fihealth.org.uk

## Haven Centre

*A national charity dedicated to providing a network of support centres for people affected by breast cancer. Havens (in London and Hereford) offer information, advice, counselling and complementary therapies under one roof, free of charge and designed to complement conventional medical treatment.*
**Address** Effie Road, Fulham Broadway, London SW6 1TB
**Tel** 020 7384 0000 **Fax** 020 7384 0001
**Email** info@breastcancerhaven.org.uk **Website** www.thehaventrust.org.uk

## Help Adolescents With Cancer

*Offers counselling, group meetings and support for families and siblings. Also holds an annual 10-day workshop/holiday in Jersey for 25-30 teenagers.*
**Address** 1st floor, Post Office Buildings, 338 Hollinwood Avenue,
New Moston, Manchester M40 0GB
**Tel** 0161 688 6244 **Fax** 0161 682 4020
**Email** niki@hawc.fsnet.co.uk **Website** www.hawc-co-uk.com

## Hospice Information

*Publishes a directory of hospice and palliative care services. For directory or details*

*of local services, send a large sae with three first-class stamps, or telephone.*
**Address** St Christopher's Hospice, 51-59 Lawrie Park Road, Sydenham,
London SE26 6DZ
**Tel** 0870 903 3903  **Fax** 020 7278 2101
**Email** info@hospiceinformation.info
**Website** www.hospiceinformation.info

### Let's Face It
*A contact point for people of any age coping with facial disfigurement, specialising in facial cancer. Telephone and letter contact, one-to-one counselling, meetings for self-help or social contact.*
**Address** 72 Victoria Avenue, Westgate-on-Sea, Kent CT8 8BH
**Tel** 01843 833724
**Email** chrisletsfaceit@aol.com  **Website** www.lets-face-it.org.uk

### Leukaemia Care
*Promotes the welfare of people with leukaemia and allied blood disorders. Offers family caravan holidays, friendships and support. Discretionary financial assistance, newsletter and publications available.*
**Address** 2 Shrubbery Avenue, Worcester WR1 1QH
**Tel** 01905 330003  **Careline** 0800 169 6680  **Fax** 01905 330090
**Email** enquiries@leukaemiacare.org.uk  **Website** www.leukaemiacare.org.uk

### Lymphoedema Support Network
*Runs a telephone helpline, produces a quarterly newsletter and a wide range of factsheets, and maintains an up-to-date website. Works to raise awareness of lymphoedema and campaigns for better national standards of care.*
**Address** St. Luke's Crypt, Sydney Street, London SW3 6NH
**Tel** Infoline 020 7351 4480  **Fax** 020 7349 9809
**E-mail** lymphoedema@freeserve.org.uk
**Website** www.lymphoedema.org/lsn

### Lymphoma Association
*Information and emotional support for lymphoma (Hodgkin's disease and non-Hodgkin's lymphoma) patients and their families. Literature, a quarterly newsletter and videos, plus a network of helpers with experience of the disease. Local groups in some areas.*

**Address** PO Box 386, Aylesbury, Bucks HP20 2GA
**Tel** 01296 619400  **Helpline** 0808 808 5555 (Mon-Fri, 9am-5pm)
**Fax** 01296 619414
**E-mail** support@lymphoma.org.uk  **Website** www.lymphoma.org.uk

## Marie Curie Cancer Care

*Hands-on palliative nursing care is provided during the day and overnight in patients' homes by a nationwide network of Marie Curie nurses. Contact the local district nursing service. Ten Marie Curie Centres, admission by referral from GP or consultant. Both services are free of charge.*
**Address** 89 Albert Embankment, London SE1 7TP
**Tel** 020 7599 7777  **Fax** 020 7599 7788
**Email** info@mariecurie.org.uk  **Website** www.mariecurie.org.uk

## National Association of Laryngectomee Clubs

*Promotes the welfare of laryngectomees. Encourages the formation of clubs to assist rehabilitation through speech therapy, social support and monthly meetings. Advises on speech aids and medical supplies. Offers referral service.*
**Address** Ground Floor, 6 Rickett Street, Fulham, London SW6 1RU
**Tel** 020 7381 9993  **Fax** 020 7381 0025
**Website** www.nalc.ik.com

## National Cancer Alliance

*Aims to represent the interests of cancer patients and their carers; to increase awareness about cancer services, diagnosis, treatment and care; to promote and monitor standards of cancer treatment and care.*
**Address** PO Box 579, Oxford OX4 1LB
**Tel** 01865 793566  **Fax** 01865 251050
**Email** nationalcanceralliance@btinternet.com
**Website** www.nationalcanceralliance.co.uk

## Natural Death Centre

*Aims to improve the quality of dying, and to help people arrange inexpensive, family-organised and environmentally friendly funerals.*
**Address** 6 Blackstock Mews, Blackstock Road, London N4 2BT
**Tel** 0871 288 2098  **Fax** 020 7354 3831
**Website** www.naturaldeath.org.uk

### Neuroblastoma Society

*Information and advice by telephone or letter for patients and their families. Provides contact where possible with others who have experienced the illness in the family, for mutual support.*

**Address** 18 Harlesden Road, St Albans,
Hertfordshire AL1 4LF
**Tel** 01727 851818 **Fax** 01727 851818
**Email** info@nsoc.co.uk **Website** www.nsoc.co.uk

### NHS Direct

*The National Health Service information service.*
**Freephone information lines** 0845 4647 (in England and Wales);
0845 4 24 24 24 (NHS 24 in Scotland)
**Website** www.nhsdirect.nhs.uk; www.nhs24.com (in Scotland)

### NICE (National Institute for Health and Clinical Excellence)

*Independent organisation responsible for providing national guidance on best practice and treatment strategies.*

**Address** MidCity Place, 71 High Holborn,
London, WC1V 6NA
**Tel** 020 7067 5800 **Fax** 020 7067 5801
**Email** nice@nice.org.uk **Website** www.nice.org.uk

### Oesophageal Patients Association

*Leaflets, telephone advice and support, before, during and after treatment. Contact where possible by former patients to people with oesophageal cancer.*

**Address** 22 Vulcan House, Vulcan Road, Solihull B91 2JY
**Tel/Fax** 0121 704 9860
**E-mail** opa@ukgateway.net **Website** www.opa.org.uk

### Ovacome

*A support organisation for people affected by ovarian cancer.*
**Address** Elizabeth Garrett Anderson Hospital, Huntley Street,
London WC2E 6DH
**Tel** 020 7380 9589
**E-mail** ovacome@ovacome.org.uk **Website** www.ovacome.org.uk

## Patients Association

*Helpline provides information on a wide range of issues, from finding local support groups to making a complaint or drawing up a living will.*
**Address** PO Box 935, Harrow, Middlesex HA1 3YJ
**Helpline** 08456 08 4455 (Mon-Fri, 10am-4pm)
**Tel** 020 8423 9111  **Fax** 020 8423 9119
**Website** www.patients-association.com

## Prostate Cancer Charity

*Aims to improve the care and welfare of people whose lives are affected by prostate cancer. Free information leaflets and telephone helpline staffed by trained nurses. Nationwide network of support contacts.*
**Address** 3 Angel Walk, Hammersmith, London W6 9HX
**Helpline** 0845 300 8383 (Mon-Fri, 10am-4pm)
**Fax** 020 8222 7634
**Email** info@prostate-cancer.org.uk  **Website** www.prostate-cancer.org.uk

## Radiotherapy Action Group Exposure (RAGE)

*A voluntary group campaigning for the needs of breast cancer patients who have suffered permanent injuries as a result of radiotherapy treatment.*
**Address** Joyce Pritchard, 24 Edgeborough Way, Bromley BR1 2UA
**Tel** 020 8460 7476  **Fax** 020 8466 7039

## Roy Castle Lung Cancer Foundation

*Dedicated to defeating lung cancer through research, prevention and support.*
**Address** 200 London Road, Liverpool L3 9TA
**Helpline** 0800 358 7200  **Tel** 0871 220 5426
**Fax** 0871 220 5427
**Email** foundation@roycastle.liv.ac.uk  **Website** www.roycastle.org

## Teenage Cancer Trust

*Provides information for teenagers and raises funds to build and equip specialist units to treat and care for adolescents with cancer, leukaemia, Hodgkin's and related diseases. Dedicated nursing posts and research into adolescent cancer.*
**Address** 38 Warren Street, London W1T 6AE
**Tel** 020 7387 1000  **Fax** 020 7387 6000
**Email** tct@teenagecancertrust.org.uk  **Website** www.teenagecancertrust.org

# BIBLIOGRAPHY

## BOOKS

Kate Carr, *It's Not Like That, Actually: a memoir of surviving cancer – and beyond*, Vermilion, 2004

John Diamond, *C: because cowards get cancer too*, Vermilion, 2004

Michael Gearin-Tosh, *Living Proof: a medical mutiny*, Scribner, 2003

Jerome E. Groopman, *The Anatomy of Hope: how people find strength in the face of illness*, Simon & Schuster, 2005

Marie de Hennezel, *Intimate Death: how the dying teach us to live*, translated by Carol Brown Janeway, Time Warner, 1998

Ruth Picardie, *Before I Say Goodbye*, Penguin, 1998

Ken Wilber, *Grace and Grit: spirituality and healing in the life of Treya Killam Wilber*, Gateway, 2001

## ARTICLES

Martyn Harris, 'This is not the time to die', *The Spectator*, 19 August 1995

Joanna Moorehead, 'I don't know what to say', *The Guardian*, G2, 8 February 2005

Penny Wark, 'A buoyant approach', *The Times*, T2, 31 January 2005

## POEMS

Julia Darling, 'How to Behave With the Ill'

Julia Darling, 'Chemotherapy'

With kind permission of Julia Darling's family to use Julia Darling's two poems, 'How to Behave With the Ill' and 'Chemotherapy' (from *Sudden Collapses in Public Places*, Arc Publications, 2003)

Deborah Hutton was a journalist for 25 years, writing for most of the country's major glossy magazines and newspapers – from *Vogue*, *Elle*, *Marie Claire* and the *Mail on Sunday*'s *You* magazine to *The Observer*, *The Guardian* and *The Sunday Times*. This was her sixth book. She lived in north London with her husband, photographer and director, Charlie Stebbings, and their four children, Archie, Romilly, Clemmie and Freddie.